ONE STOP DOC

Gastrointestinal System

One Stop Doc

Titles in the series include:

Cell and Molecular Biology – Desikan Rangarajan & David Shaw
Editorial Advisor – Barbara Moreland

Cardiovascular System – Jonathan Aron
Editorial Advisor – Jeremy Ward

Nervous System – Elliott Smock
Editorial Advisor – Clive Coen

Coming soon...

Respiratory System – Jo Dartnell and Michelle Ramsay
Editorial Advisor – John Rees

Musculoskeletal System – Bassel Zebian and Wayne Lam
Editorial Advisor – Alistair Hunter

Renal and Urinary System and Electrolyte Balance – Panos Stamoulos and Spyros Bakalis
Editorial Advisor – Richard Naftalin and Alistair Hunter

Endocrine and Reproductive Systems – Caroline Jewel and Alexandra Tillett
Editorial Advisor – Stuart Milligan

Nutrition and Metabolism – Miruna Canagaratnam and David Shaw
Editorial Advisor – Barbara Moreland and Richard Naftalin

ONE STOP DOC

Gastrointestinal System

Miruna Canagaratnam BSc(Hons)
Fourth year medical student, Guy's, King's and
St Thomas' Medical School, London, UK

Editorial Advisor: Richard J Naftalin MB CHB MSc PHD DSc
Professor of Epithelial Physiology, King's College London Guy's
Campus Centre for Vascular Biology and Medicine, London, UK

Series Editor: Elliott Smock BSc(Hons)
Fifth year medical student, Guy's, King's and
St Thomas' Medical School, London, UK

ARNOLD

A member of the Hodder Headline Group
LONDON

First published in Great Britain in 2004 by
Arnold, a member of the Hodder Headline Group,
338 Euston Road, London NW1 3BH

http://www.arnoldpublishers.com

Distributed in the United States of America by
Oxford University Press Inc.,
198 Madison Avenue, New York, NY10016
Oxford is a registered trademark of Oxford University Press

Whilst the advice and information in this book are believed to be true and
accurate at the date of going to press, neither the authors nor the publisher
can accept any legal responsibility or liability for any errors or omissions
that may be made. In particular (but without limiting the generality of the
preceding disclaimer) every effort has been made to check drug dosages;
however it is still possible that errors have been missed. Furthermore,
dosage schedules are constantly being revised and new side-effects
recognized. For these reasons the reader is strongly urged to consult the
drug companies' printed instructions before administering any of the drugs
recommended in this book.

British Library Cataloguing in Publication Data
A catalogue record for this book is available from the British Library

Library of Congress Cataloging-in-Publication Data
A catalog record for this book is available from the Library of Congress

ISBN 10: 0 340 813431
ISBN 13: 978 0 340 813430

2 3 4 5 6 7 8 9 10

Commissioning Editor: Georgina Bentliff
Project Editor: Heather Smith
Production Controller: Lindsay Smith
Cover Design: Amina Dudhia

Typeset in 10/12pt Adobe Garamond/Akzidenz GroteskBE by Servis Filmsetting Ltd, Manchester
Printed and bound in Spain

Hodder Headline's policy is to use papers that are natural, renewable and recyclable products
and made from wood grown in sustainable forests. The logging and manufacturing processes
are expected to conform to the environmental regulations of the country of origin.

What do you think about this book? Or any other Arnold title?
Please send your comments to **feedback.arnold@hodder.co.uk**

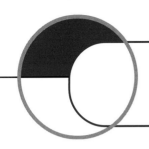

CONTENTS

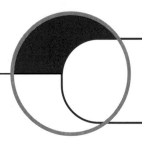

PREFACE

From the Series Editor, Elliott Smock

Are you ready to face your looming exams? If you have done loads of work, then congratulations; we hope this opportunity to practise SAQs, EMQs, MCQs and Problem-based Questions on every part of the core curriculum will help you consolidate what you've learnt and improve your exam technique. If you don't feel ready, don't panic – the One Stop Doc series has all the answers you need to catch up and pass.

There are only a limited number of questions an examiner can throw at a beleaguered student and this text can turn that to your advantage. By getting straight into the heart of the core questions that come up year after year and by giving you the model answers you need this book will arm you with the knowledge to succeed in your exams. Broken down into logical sections, you can learn all the important facts you need to pass without having to wade through tons of different textbooks when you simply don't have the time. All questions presented here are 'core'; those of the highest importance have been highlighted to allow even sharper focus if time for revision is running out. In addition, to allow you to organize your revision efficiently, questions have been grouped by topic, with answers supported by detailed integrated explanations.

On behalf of all the One Stop Doc authors I wish you the very best of luck in your exams and hope these books serve you well!

From the Author, Miruna Canagaratnam

The gastrointestinal system is **not** boring, daunting, or complicated, but can be fascinating, clear-cut and painless to learn about – and this book will you show you how.

It is divided into three chapters based on the anatomy of the gastrointestinal tract. Each chapter covers the normal development, anatomy, physiology and pharmacology of the system, focusing on the fundamentals of what you **will be tested on** in exams. In addition it covers common pathology of the gut, for those hoping to broaden their knowledge and impress their tutors ahead of the clinical years!

I'd like to extend my heartfelt thanks to Professor Richard Naftalin, who has been an invaluable source of information, constructive criticism and support. Every fact and figure has been checked, double-checked and then triple-checked by him. Without his hard work, enthusiasm, and attention to detail it would not have been possible to produce this book. I'd also like to thank Elliott for giving me the opportunity to do what I love best: write, and also for trusting me to do the job.

I would like to dedicate this book to my mum and dad.

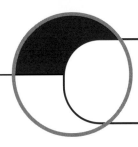

ABBREVIATIONS

ACh	acetylcholine
ALT	alanine aminotransferase
APUD	amine precursor uptake and decarboxylation
AST	aspartate aminotransferase
ATP	adenosine triphosphate
cAMP	cyclic adenosine monophosphate
CCK	cholecystokinin
COX	cyclooxygenase
DD	duodenum
ECF	extracellular fluid
GB	gallbladder

GFR	glomerular filtration rate
GGT	gamma glutamyl transferase
GI	gastrointestinal
GIP	gastrointestinal inhibitory peptide
IP_3	inositol triphosphate
i.v.	intravenous
IVC	inferior vena cava
MALT	mucosal-associated lymphoid tissue
NSAID	non-steroidal anti-inflammatory drug
PGE_2	prostaglandin E_2
RBC	red blood cell
sER	smooth endoplasmic reticulum

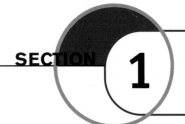

UPPER GASTROINTESTINAL TRACT

 1. Is it true or false that in the salivon (the functional subunit of the salivary gland)

    a. Na^+ is passively reabsorbed in the excretory duct
    b. The primary secretion is hypotonic to plasma
    c. The composition of the saliva depends on its flow rate
    d. The pH of saliva depends on its flow rate
    e. Parasympathetic stimulation produces a thick mucoid secretion

2. Consider the salivon below

    a. List the functions of salivation
    b. Label the parts of the salivon indicated in the diagram below

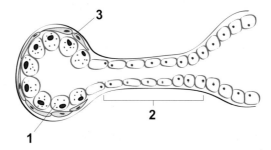

3. Saliva secretion

    a. Occurs only on stimulation of the sublingual gland
    b. May increase by 15 times if food is present in the mouth
    c. Can be stimulated by smell
    d. Decreases at night
    e. Is an unconditioned reflex

EXPLANATION: SALIVA

Saliva has several functions in the oral cavity **(2a)**:

- It contains mucins, glycoproteins which provide **lubrication** to assist swallowing
- It **moistens mouth** and **tongue** to facilitate speech
- It contains **IgA**, the first defence against bacteria and viruses, as well as **lysozyme**, which attacks bacterial walls
- It initiates **digestion**: salivary alpha-amylase hydrolyses starch, lingual lipase breaks down triglycerides
- It is **alkaline** to buffer mouth acid and maintain oral pH at 7.0, and also to prevent Na^+ ion loss.

Saliva is secreted by **acinar** cells, which make up units called **salivons**. On secretion it is isotonic to plasma. It then undergoes secondary modification in the intercalated and excretory ducts. Na^+ is actively reabsorbed and Cl^- is passively taken up with it. K^+ and HCO_3^- are actively secreted into the ducts. Saliva therefore reaches the end of the duct, **hypotonic** to plasma (200 mosmol/L) and alkaline.

There are **three pairs** of salivary glands in the human.

Gland	Type	Secretion
Parotid	Serous	Watery
Submandibular	Mixed	Moderately viscous
Sublingual	Mucous	Viscous

The **parotids** and **submandibular** glands secrete on stimulation, but the **sublingual** gland secretes a thin watery fluid all the time at a rate of about 0.5 mL/min. Around 1500 mL of saliva are secreted every 24 hours. Saliva contains amylase, ribonuclease, R protein, lipase, lysozyme, IgA, IgG and IgM. **Myoepithelial cells** contract around acini in response to stimuli to cause extrusion of fluid from zymogen granules inside the cells.

The composition of saliva varies with flow rate: increasing flow, increases salivary Na^+ and Cl^- concentration, because there is less time for ion reabsorption. At low flows, saliva is rich in K^+ but depleted of Na^+ and Cl^-. The presence of anything in the mouth (not necessarily food!) will stimulate saliva secretion. **Parasympathetic** cholinergic stimulation produces **watery secretion**, and can be blocked by atropine and other anticholinergic agents. **Sympathetic** adrenergic or noradrenergic stimulation produces **mucus secretion**.

Answers
1. F F T T F
2. a. See explanation. b. 1 – acinus cell; 2 – intercalated excretory duct; 3 – myoepithelial cell
3. F T T T T

4. Concerning the anatomy of the oral cavity

a. It is divided into the vestibule and the mouth proper
b. The soft palate moves away from the wall of the pharynx during swallowing
c. All the muscles of the tongue are supplied by the hypoglossal nerve
d. General sensation to the anterior two-thirds of the tongue is supplied by the lingual nerve
e. The tonsils lie posterior to both the palatoglossal and palatopharangeal arches

5. Regarding the tongue

a. Extrinsic muscles control its movement
b. It is attached to the floor of the mouth by the remnants of the thyroglossal duct
c. Vallate papillae lie anterior to sulcus terminalis
d. Section of the hypoglossal nerve causes deviation of the tongue towards the paralysed side
e. The chorda tympani supplies taste to the anterior two-thirds of the tongue

6. Concerning the muscles of mastication

a. They are innervated by the fifth cranial nerve (trigeminal)
b. Buccinator is the principal muscle used in mastication
c. Masseter originates from the zygomatic arch
d. Lateral pterygoids act together to elevate the mandible
e. Medial pterygoids produce a grinding motion

EXPLANATION: THE ORAL CAVITY

The oral cavity consists of the **vestibule** and the **mouth** proper. The roof is formed by the palate, and posteriorly the oral cavity communicates with the oropharynx. The **oropharynx** is bounded by the **soft palate** above, the epiglottis below and the palatoglossal arches laterally.

Muscles of the soft palate arise from the base of the skull. They are **levator veli palatine, tensor veli palatini, palatoglossus, palatopharangeus** and **muscularis uvulae**. The tonsils lie between the arches formed by palatopharangeus and palatoglossus.

The tongue is divided in half by the lingual septum. In each half there are four extrinsic muscles and four intrinsic muscles. The tongue is attached to the floor of the mouth by the **lingual frenulum** on its underside. If you lift up your tongue the lingual veins running on either side of the frenulum can be seen.

All the muscles of the tongue except palatoglossus are innervated by the **hypoglossal nerve** (XII). Section of the hypoglossal nerve results in paralysis and atrophy of one side of the tongue. The tongue deviates to the paralysed side when it is stuck out because of the unopposed action of the unaffected genioglossus muscle on the other side.

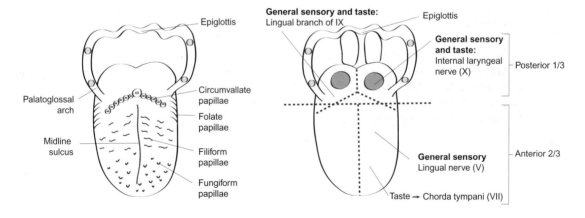

Movement of the temporal mandibular joint is mainly achieved by the muscles of mastication: **temporalis, masseter, medial pterygoid**, which produce the biting motion, and **lateral pterygoid** which protudes the mandible.

Answers
4. T F F T F
5. T F T T T
6. T F T F T

7. Arrange the following statements in chronological order

A. Elevation of the larynx
B. Relaxation of the upper oesophageal sphincter
C. Primary wave of peristalsis down the oesophagus
D. Mastication of food
E. Involuntary contraction of pharynx walls
F. Elevation of soft palate
G. Tongue raised against hard palate

8. True or false? Swallowing

a. Has four phases
b. Can be stopped once initiated
c. Is coordinated by the swallowing centre in the medulla
d. Is initiated by the tongue
e. Results in choking if the glottis is not closed

9. Regarding the pharynx, which of the following statements are true?

a. It is a common route for both food and air
b. It has three constrictor muscles
c. It constricts to prevent passage of food
d. The pharangeal plexus is formed from the branches of the eighth and ninth nerves
e. It is not involved in voice production

EXPLANATION: SWALLOWING

The **pharynx** is a funnel-shaped tube of muscle that conducts food to the oesophagus and air to the larynx. It is about 15 cm long and extends from the base of the skull to the inferior border of C6 vertebra. The pharynx consists of three constrictor muscles: the superior, middle and inferior muscles, which overlap one another. It also has three other muscles which descend from the styloid process (stylopharangeus), the cartilaginous part of the auditory tube (salpingopharynegeus), and the soft palate (palatopharyngeus).

The **three constrictors** constrict the wall of the pharynx during **swallowing**, the other **three muscles elevate** the pharynx and larynx during **swallowing** and **speaking**.

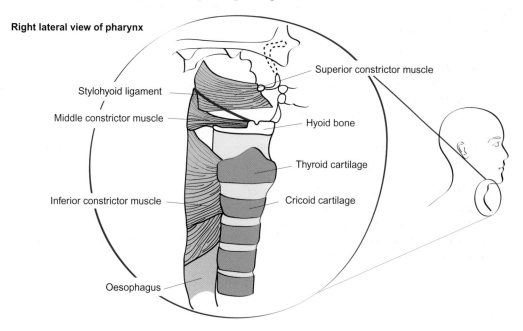

Right lateral view of pharynx

Stylohyoid ligament
Middle constrictor muscle
Inferior constrictor muscle
Oesophagus
Superior constrictor muscle
Hyoid bone
Thyroid cartilage
Cricoid cartilage

Swallowing has an initial **voluntary phase** followed by a second **involuntary phase**. In the first stage a decision is made to swallow. Food that has been chewed (masticated) is combined with saliva to form a bolus and pushed to the oropharynx by the tongue. The tongue presses against the hard palate. The soft palate is elevated to prevent food entering the nasopharynx.

In the second stage there is a reflex relaxation of the upper oesophageal sphincter and the walls of the pharynx constrict to push the bolus down the pharynx into the oesophagus. The contraction of these muscles raises the pharynx and the larynx. Both respiration and chewing stop during swallowing. The **epiglottis reflexively closes** to prevent food entering the **larynx**.

Answers
7. 1 – D, 2 – G, 3 – F, 4 – B, 5 – E, 6 – A, 7 – C
8. F F T T T
9. T T F F F

10. Concerning the development of the digestive system

   a. The primitive gut tube forms in the fourth week
   b. The mesenchyme gives rise to the epithelium of the gastrointestinal tract
   c. The primitive gut is divided into three parts
   d. The ventral part of the yolk sac is incorporated into the gut tube
   e. Connective tissue and muscle are formed from the endoderm

11. Regarding development of the oesophagus

   a. The oesophagus reaches its final relative length by week 7 of embryonic development
   b. The oesophagus is separated from the laryngotracheal tube by the tracheoesophageal septum
   c. The glands of the oesophagus are derived from the endoderm
   d. Smooth muscle develops from the splanchnic mesenchyme
   e. Oesophageal atresia is caused by hypertrophy of the striated muscle from the branchial arches

12. True or false? The stomach

   a. Does not develop until the eighth week
   b. Is attached to the liver by the dorsal mesentery
   c. Grows faster dorsally than ventrally
   d. Is continually orientated in the median plane
   e. Is supplied from the coeliac trunk

GI, gastrointestinal

EXPLANATION: DEVELOPMENT OF THE DIGESTIVE SYSTEM

The trilaminar embryonic disc that is formed in the **third week** of human development consists of three germ cell layers: the **ectoderm**, **mesoderm** and **endoderm**. As the embryo develops, these layers give rise to the tissues and organs of the embryo.

In the fourth week, folding of the embryo in median and horizontal planes converts the flat embryonic disc into a C-shaped cylindrical embryo with a head and tail. The primitive gut tube emerges from the dorsal part of the yolk sac with this sequence of folding events. It is divided into **foregut**, **midgut** and **hindgut**.

The **endoderm** of the primitive gut tube gives rise to the **epithelium** of the GI tract as well as the parenchyma of the associated glands: the liver and pancreas. The splanchnic **mesenchyme** that surrounds the endoderm gives rise to the **connective tissue** and **muscles** of the tract.

The oesophagus lengthens as a result of cranial body growth, and is usually at its final length by seven weeks. The **striated muscle** that makes up the upper third of the oesophagus is formed from the mesenchyme of the caudal branchial arches. The **smooth muscle** of the lower two-thirds of the oesophagus is derived from the splanchnic mesenchyme.

Oesophageal atresia is a developmental abnormality that results from abnormal deviation of the tracheoe-sophageal septum in a posterior direction, where there is incomplete separation of the laryngotracheal tube from the oesophagus.

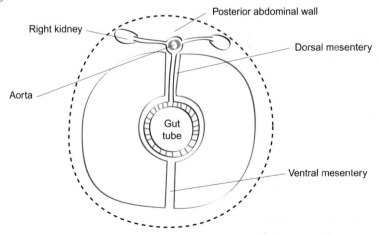

The stomach forms from a local dilation in the gut tube in the fourth week as shown in the above cross-section. It is suspended from the dorsal wall of the abdominal cavity by a **dorsal mesentery** and attached to the liver and ventral abdominal wall by a **ventral mesentery**.

Answers
10. T F T F F
11. T F T T F
12. F F T F T

13. On the diagram below of the developing stomach at six weeks, label the following

Options

A. Aorta
B. Dilation of foregut
C. Dorsal mesentery
D. Ventral mesentery

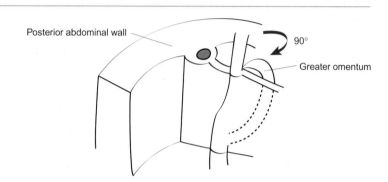

14. Concerning peritoneal coverings

a. The parietal peritoneum is held against the abdominal wall by the intra-abdominal fascia
b. The peritoneal cavity contains air only
c. Organs between the visceral and parietal peritoneum are termed retroperitoneal
d. The lesser sac lies behind the stomach
e. The greater omentum is fused to the transverse mesocolon

15. The following organs are retroperitoneal

a. Kidneys
b. Liver
c. Pancreas
d. Duodenum
e. Stomach

16. True or false? Pyloric stenosis

a. Affects 1 in 150 infants
b. Is caused by hypertrophy of the pylorus
c. Causes projectile vomiting
d. Can be felt as an enlarged mass in the right upper quadrant
e. Is untreatable

EXPLANATION: THE STOMACH

The stomach tends to enlarge and broaden over the fifth and sixth weeks. It grows faster dorsally than ventrally, giving it its characteristic shape and demarcating the greater curvature.

As shown below, the stomach **rotates** about its longitudinal axis, **90° clockwise**, so that the left side faces anteriorly and the right side posteriorly.

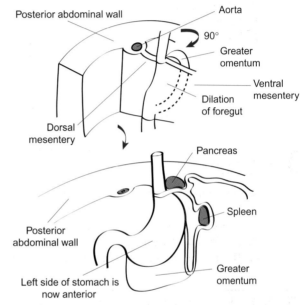

Since the mesenteries also rotate with the stomach, there is formation of the greater omentum by the dorsal mesentery, and the omental bursa or lesser sac posterior to the stomach. The lesser sac communicates with the main part of the peritoneal cavity through the epiploic foramen.

Congenital pyloric stenosis affects 1 in 150 male infants and 1 in 750 females. It is caused by hypertrophy of the circular muscles of the pylorus in the stomach. This narrowing obstructs flow of food from the stomach to the duodenum, and results in projectile vomiting, without bile. The enlarged pylorus can be felt in the right upper quadrant. It is usually treated by surgery.

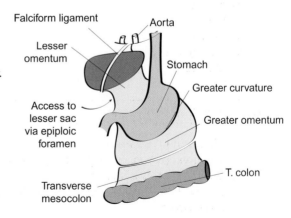

Answers
13. See explanation
14. T F F T T
15. T F T T F
16. F T T T F

17. Describe how the following contribute to the pathogenesis of peptic ulceration

    a. *Helicobacter pylori*
    b. Aspirin

18. Case study

A 46-year-old man is admitted to hospital with a 3-day history of sharp stomach pains and an episode of vomiting blood. For the past two weeks he has been taking aspirin for a back injury. On examination in the Emergency Department he was observed to be pale and tachycardic with a low blood pressure. He was provisionally diagnosed with a gastric ulcer.
    a. What may have caused the man to vomit blood?
    b. How should he be treated?
    c. How might this be prevented from happening again?

19. True or false? *Helicobacter pylori*

    a. Is a gram-positive bacillus
    b. Requires a pH lower than 3 for optimum growth
    c. Is strongly associated with chronic gastritis
    d. Secretes myeloperoxidase which destroys epithelial cells
    e. May be eradicated by standard triple therapy

NSAID, non-steroidal anti-inflammatory drug; COX, cyclooxygenase; PGE$_2$, prostaglandin E$_2$; i.v., intravenous

EXPLANATION: PEPTIC ULCERS

Helicobacter pylori is a **gram-negative** spiral-shaped bacteria which colonizes the gastric mucosa, most commonly in the antrum of the stomach. It is present in 70 per cent of patients with gastric peptic ulcers and almost all patients with duodenal peptic ulcers. It is also present in 90 per cent of chronic active gastritis cases. Antibiotic treatment of *H. pylori* promotes the healing of ulcers and prevents their recurrence.
It is thought that *H. pylori* impairs mucosal defenses by:

- Secreting a protease that breaks down glycoproteins in gastric mucosa
- Producing phospholipases which damage epithelial cells
- Secreting a urease that generates free ammonia.

Neutrophils attracted to *H. pylori* release myeloperoxidase, which produces monochloramine in the presence of ammonia. Monochloramine destroys cells **(17a)**.

Due to **intracellular urease activity** the internal pH in **H. pylori** is buffered to neutral when the external pH falls below 3.

Aspirin is an NSAID that causes irreversible inhibition of **cyclooxygenase** by acetylating a serine residue at its active site. Therefore the production of prostaglandins by the COX pathway is inhibited. PGE_2 acts on parietal cells to inhibit acid secretion into the gastric lumen. Removal of this inhibition **encourages acid secretion,** which in turn causes gastric irritation, leading to a **peptic ulcer (17b)**. People who take low doses of aspirin for long periods to prevent myocardial infarction, unstable angina and stroke are at **risk for peptic ulcers**.

Peptic ulceration is the erosion of a small solitary patch of the stomach or duodenum lining due to exposure to acid peptic juices. The man in our case study is likely to have a peptic ulcer which has **bled**, causing him to experience pain and vomit **(18a)**. This man is suffering from hypovolaemic shock – hence the need for resuscitation and fluids. Treatment would involve **(18b)** resuscitation with i.v. saline or colloids, an **H₂ antagonist** (cimetidine) or **proton pump inhibitor** (omeprazole), a urea breath test for *H. pylori*, which can be eradicated with triple therapy, stopping the aspirin and giving an alternative pain killer for back pain, and finally **lifestyle advice** (reduce stress, stop smoking) **(18c)**.

Answers
17. See explanation
18. See explanation
19. F F T F T

20. **The following factors either (1) increase acid secretion or (2) impair mucosal defenses. Label them accordingly**

Options

    A. Alcohol
    B. Caffeine
    C. Anticancer drugs
    D. Stress
    E. Hyperparathyroidism
    F. Smoking

21. **Describe briefly the mechanism of action of the following drugs used to inhibit gastric acid secretion and give the class of each drug**

    a. Magnesium hydroxide
    b. Ranitidine
    c. Omeprazole

EXPLANATION: GASTRIC ACID SECRETION

We become predisposed to conditions such as **peptic ulceration**, **reflux oesophagitis** and **gastritis** if there is a chronic increase in acid secretion by parietal cells and/or an impairment in mucosal protection.

A **peptic ulcer** is the **commonest** cause of **bleeding** from the upper GI tract. It may be acute and severe enough to cause hypovolaemic shock. Ingestion of NSAIDs, steroids or anticoagulants also predisposes to bleeding.

Causes of increased acid secretion	Causes of mucosal barrier breakdown
Caffeine – stimulates cAMP activation	Alcohol, vinegar and bile salts disrupt the unstirred layer
Smoking	NSAIDs, e.g. aspirin, disrupt the unstirred layer and inhibit PG synthesis
Zollinger–Ellison syndrome – characterized by gastrin-secreting adenomas	Anticancer drugs – reduced regeneration of epithelial cells
Hyperparathyroidism – raised plasma Ca levels stimulate acid secretion	*H. pylori* – a gram-negative bacterium that colonizes gastric mucosa
Stress	

Salts of magnesium/aluminium are commonly known as **antacids**. Taken orally they act to neutralize gastric acid and raise gastric pH **(21a)**. Ranitidine belongs to a group of drugs called histamine receptor antagonists. It inhibits histamine-stimulated acid secretion by **parietal cells** in the gastric mucosa **(21b)**.

Parietal cells have H_2 **receptors** on their cell surface membranes which when activated stimulate adenylate cyclase to produce **cAMP** which in turn activates a protein kinase cascade, ending in stimulation of a proton pump at the luminal surface of the cell. Inhibition of these receptors causes a decrease in the production of cAMP, resulting in a decrease in the activity of the H^+/K^+ ATPase (proton pump). Therefore less acid is secreted into the stomach lumen.

Omeprazole is an **irreversible proton pump inhibitor**. This drug is activated at a pH lower than 3 to form a disulphide link with the H^+/K^+ ATPase, which directly blocks the pump, reducing H^+ ion secretion into the lumen **(21c)**.

Answers
20. 1 – B, D, E, F; 2 – A, C
21. See explanation

22. The following are symptoms of peptic ulceration. True or false?

a. Abdominal pain after eating
b. Nausea
c. Vomiting of blood
d. Water brash
e. Diarrhoea

23. Theme – pharmacology of peptic ulcers. Match the following drugs with the mechanisms of action listed below

Options

A. Omeprazole
B. Cimetidine
C. Pirenzipine
D. Magnesium hydroxide
E. Bismuth chelate
F. Misoprostol

1. Analogue of prostaglandin E_1 to inhibit gastric acid secretion
2. Histamine receptor blockade
3. Coats gastric mucosa and eradicates *H. pylori*
4. Proton pump inhibition
5. Neutralizes gastric acid
6. Muscarinic receptor blockade on parietal cells

EXPLANATION: PEPTIC ULCERS – SYMPTOMS AND TREATMENT

Symptoms of peptic ulceration include:

- Abdominal pain which gets worse at night but is relieved by food
- Nausea and vomiting (may contain blood)
- Poor sleep

In treating peptic ulceration, the general principles are to **relieve pain**, **heal mucosa** and **prevent relapse**. *H. pylori* can be eliminated using **triple therapy**: two antibiotics and a proton pump inhibitor (e.g. amoxycillin, metronidazole and omeprazole).

	Antacids	H$_2$ Histamine antagonists	Proton pump inhibitors	Muscarinic receptor antagonists
Taken	Orally	Orally	Orally but enteric coated granules in capsule	Orally
Action	Neutralize gastric acid, raise pH. Inhibit peptic activity	Block action of Histamine on parietal cells. Reduce acid secretion	Block the H$^+$/K$^+$ ATPase pump irreversibly. Reduce acid secretion	Block action of ACh on parietal cells. Reduce acid secretion and motility
Example	Salts of Mg^{2+}, Al^{3+}	Cimetidine, ranitidine	Omeprazole, lansoprazole	Pirenzipine
Side effects	Mg^{2+} – diarrhoea Al^{3+} – constipation Acid rebound is a side effect of antacids	Rarely anti-androgenic, gynaecomastia. Reduce hepatic metabolism of other diagnoses	Rare headache, diarrhoea, rashes	Dry mouth, blurred vision (in 20% of patients)
Effect on ulcers	High doses promote ulcer healing	Relieve pain of ulcer and increase rate of ulcer healing	Particularly useful for severe ulceration resistant to other drugs	As effective as cimetidine but side effects common

Answers
22. F T T T F
23. 1 – F, 2 – B, 3 – E, 4 – A, 5 – D, 6 – C

24. Sketch a graph to show the three phases of gastric acid secretion that follow feeding. Indicate the stimulus necessary to initiate each phase

25. Concerning gastric secretions

    a. The pylorus is the major secretory region in the stomach
    b. Chief cells lie deep within the gastric glands
    c. The acid provides optimum conditions for proteolytic enzyme activity
    d. Intrinsic factor is not a necessary component of gastric secretion
    e. The stomach only secretes gastric juice on stimulation

26. True or false? Gastrin

    a. Is a 17 amino acid chain
    b. Is secreted by parietal cells
    c. Secretion is stimulated by caffeine
    d. May be stimulated by local distension of the antrum
    e. May be produced by certain tumours

ACh, acetylcholine; IP$_3$, inositol triphosphate; cAMP, cyclic adenosine monophosphate; GIP, gastrointestinal inhibitory peptide; CCK, cholecystokinin

EXPLANATION: GASTRIC SECRETIONS

On average, the gastric glands of the stomach produce 2–3 L of gastric juice per day, largely made up of **hydrochloric acid**, **pepsinogens** and **intrinsic factor**. The fundus and the antrum are the main secretory regions of the stomach.

Hydrochloric acid produced by the parietal cells, also called oxyntic cells, has the following actions:

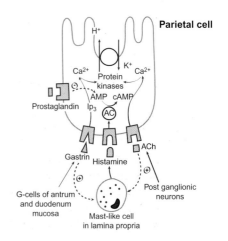

Parietal cell

- Kills many ingested bacteria
- Lowers the pH to activate pepsin which starts protein digestion
- Aids protein digestion
- Stimulates flow of bile and pancreatic juice.

Acid is secreted from parietal cells (see diagram) via a **proton pump**. Acid secretion by the cells is stimulated by three main factors:

- Gastrin (a peptide hormone)
- ACh (a neurotransmitter)
- Histamine (a local hormone).

The diagram below shows the three phases of gastric acid secretion **(24)**.

1. CEPHALIC PHASE   Food in mouth reflexly stimulates gastric acid secretion via efferent fibres of the vagus nerve. ACh acts directly on parietal cells as well as G-cells in the antrum and duodenum to release gastrin, and on mast-like cells to release histamine.

2. GASTRIC PHASE   Presence of food in the stomach causes distension. This causes mechanoreceptors to initiate a reflex cholinergic response. Amino acids or peptides act directly on G-cells in the antrum to release gastrin.

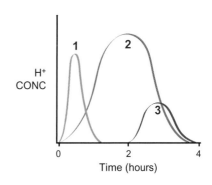

3. INTESTINAL PHASE   Presence of chyme in the duodenum above pH 3 causes gastrin release. Presence of chyme in the duodenum below pH 2 causes secretin release, which inhibits gastrin secretion. Fatty acids cause release of GIP and CCK, both of which depress acid secretion by parietal cells.

Answers
24. See explanation
25. F T T F F
26. T F T T T

27. True or false? Hiatus hernias

a. Are caused by the stomach riding up through the oesophageal hiatus
b. Result in regurgitation of food
c. May lead to a painful shoulder
d. Are associated with an increased risk of oesophageal carcinoma
e. Are common in young children

28. Case study

A 55-year-old man presents to the Emergency Department with a two-week history of retrosternal chest pain, which comes on after eating, lying down or bending over. He also complains of excess saliva in his mouth, and occasional difficulty swallowing. An ECG and X-rays of the abdomen are ordered.

a. What is a hiatus hernia?
b. What investigation must be carried out to confirm the diagnosis?
c. How may this patient be treated?

29. True or false? The oesophagus

a. Lies posterior to the trachea in the superior mediastinum
b. Is compressed by the arch of the aorta
c. Pierces the diaphragm at the level of T12
d. Contains involuntary muscle in its upper third
e. Inclines to the right

30. Achalasia

a. Is caused by degeneration of the vagus nerve
b. Results in a chronically contracted lower oesophageal sphincter
c. Is virtually indistinguishable from Chagas' disease
d. Causes dysphagia
e. Causes hyperpropulsive peristalsis

EXPLANATION: THE OESOPHAGUS AND HIATUS HERNIA

The oesophagus is divided into **cervical**, **thoracic** and **abdominal** parts. It enters the superior mediastinum between the trachea and vertebral column. Behind the trachea it inclines to the left so that it lies behind the left bronchus in the posterior mediastinum. In its descent to the diaphragm, however, it crosses in front of the descending aorta to the midline. It pierces the diaphragm at the level of **T10**. The muscle of the oesophagus is **voluntary** in its upper third, and **involuntary** in its lower two-thirds.

1. SLIDING - Abdominal part of oesophagus slides upwards

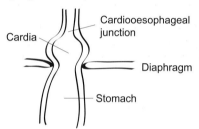

Cardia — Cardiooesophageal junction — Diaphragm — Stomach

2. PARAOESOPHAGEAL - Cardia remains in place, part of the stomach slips through the oesophages hiatus

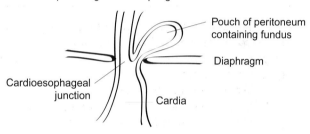

Pouch of peritoneum containing fundus — Diaphragm — Cardioesophageal junction — Cardia

Hiatus hernias may be **sliding** or **paraoesophageal**. Sliding occurs more commonly. They occur when intra-abdominal pressure is higher than intrathoracic pressure; for example, when stooping, straining, coughing or during pregnancy **(28a)**. They may also occur if the clamping action of the right crus of the diaphragm on the lower oesophagus is weak. Most people have no symptoms. However some experience reflux of food and acid, which can lead to chronic irritation and ulceration. Other symptoms are water brash (sudden salivation) and dysphagia. Referred pain to the shoulder may occur because the phrenic nerve innervates the parietal peritoneum and pleura as well as the pericardium next to the diaphragm. Pain is referred to the dermatomes of C3, 4 and 5, the skin of the neck and shoulder.

A **hiatus hernia** may be demonstrated through a **barium meal radiological examination (28b)**. Endoscopy should also be performed to assess the presence of reflux oesophagitis and also to exclude carcinoma. Symptoms may be managed non-operatively in 85 per cent of cases. Measures such as avoiding tight clothing and bending, stopping smoking and losing weight can be beneficial. Surgery may be performed if symptoms persist **(28c)**.

Achalasia is obstruction at the lower oesophageal sphincter due to a failure of relaxation. It is thought to be caused by degeneration of the ganglion cells in Auerbach's plexus. **Chagas' disease** is an infection by *Trypanosoma cruzi* which causes similar degenerative changes. The patient has difficulty swallowing (dysphagia) since motility is disordered. Peristalsis is absent.

Answers
27. T T T T F
28. See explanation
29. T T F F F
30. F T T T F

31. The following factors inhibit the feeding centre in the lateral hypothalamus in short-term feeding regulation

    a. Neuropeptide Y
    b. Chewing
    c. Insulin
    d. Amino acids
    e. Stomach distension

32. Regarding the control of food intake, are the following statements true or false?

    a. Lesion to the ventromedial hypothalamus causes hyperphagia
    b. Lesion to the lateral hypothalamus causes anorexia
    c. Glucostats increase their activity to stimulate the feeding centre
    d. Distension of the stomach is a satiety signal
    e. Cholecystokinin is a satiety signal

33. Regarding the control of body weight

    a. Leptin is secreted by enterocytes
    b. Obese people have more fat cells than people of normal weight
    c. Leptin counteracts the effects of neuropeptide Y
    d. Obese people have lower leptin levels than people of normal weight
    e. Excess leptin causes uncontrolled food intake

GI, gastrointestinal; CCK, cholecystokinin

EXPLANATION: SATIETY

The feeling of fullness or satiety after eating results from stimulation of the satiety centre in the **ventromedial hypothalamus**. Lesion to this centre causes hyperphagia. The feeding centre lies in the lateral hypothalamus. Stimulation evokes feeding, whereas destruction causes anorexia. Glucose and amino acids inhibit the feeding centre, as do chewing, swallowing and tasting. It is thought that normally the feeding centre is continuously active. Its activity is inhibited transiently by the satiety centre after feeding.

Glucostats are central cells whose glucose utilization governs the activity of the feeding centre. When blood glucose is low, the activity of these cells is decreased and therefore the activity of the feeding centre is unchecked. When blood glucose is high, the utilization by these cells is high and therefore the activity of the feeding centre is inhibited, thus the individual feels sated.

Satiety signals include stomach distension, which increases **vagal activity** via **mechanoreceptors** to inhibit appetite, and **CCK** release, which (1) slows gastric emptying to maintain gastric distension (indirect effect) and (2) reduces food intake by mimicking the vagal activity caused by gastric distension (direct effect). Smell, taste, habit conditioning, chewing and swallowing cause **satiety** even before food reaches the stomach.

Leptin is a hormone secreted by **adipocytes** (fat cells). Circulating levels are proportional to the total amount of fat in the body. Leptin acts at the **hypothalamus** to inhibit food intake. It counteracts the effects of **neuropeptide Y**. Neuropeptide Y is released by the movement of foods along the GI tract and stimulates the feeding centre. Leptin also increases fat metabolism, and increases energy expenditure.

Answers
31. F T T T F
32. T T F T F
33. F T T F F

34. Label the diagram of the GI tract below using the list provided

Options

A. Lamina propria
C. Submucosa
E. Myenteric plexus

B. Circular muscularis
D. Lumen

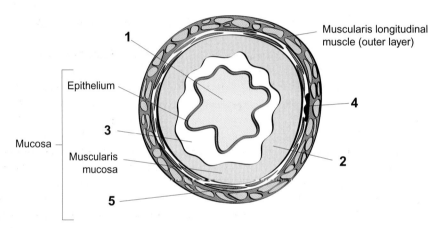

35. Theme – physiology of the GI tract. Match the histological feature of the GI tract to its function in the list below

Options

A. Parietal cell
C. Mucous cell
E. Villi
G. Goblet cell

B. Chief (zymogen) cell
D. Brunner's gland
F. APUD cell

1. Secretion of secretin and cholecystokinin
2. Pepsin secretion
3. Increased surface area for absorption
4. Secretion of acidic mucus in duodenal lumen
5. Acid secretion
6. Secretion of alkaline mucus in duodenal lumen
7. Secretion of mucus into stomach lumen

CCK, cholecystokinin; GI, gastrointestinal; APUD, amine precursor uptake and decarboxylation

EXPLANATION: PHYSIOLOGY OF THE GASTROINTESTINAL TRACT

The GI tract is essentially a **muscular tube** lined by a **mucous membrane**. The major muscular component remains relatively constant throughout the tract whereas the mucosa shows marked variations. The GI tract has four distinct layers:

- Mucosa
- Submucosa
- Muscularis: longitudinal and circular
- Adventitia.

Within the mucosa, are three sublayers: the epithelium, lamina propria and muscularis mucosa.

Large clusters of parasympathetic ganglion cells are found between the two layers of the muscularis. This is the **myenteric plexus**. Smaller clusters of parasympathetic ganglion cells in the submucosa that supply mucosal glands and the smooth muscle of the muscularis mucosae are called **Meissner's plexus**.

At different parts of the tract the mucosa changes from one form to another. The mucosa of the oral cavity, pharynx, oesophagus and anal canal is **protective**, consisting of stratified squamous cells. **Secretory** mucosa in the stomach consists of long, closely packed tubular glands that may be simple or branched.

The mucosa of the small intestine is entirely **absorptive**. The mucosa is arranged into finger-like projections called villi, with short intervening crypts. The large intestine is lined with a combination of **absorptive/protective** mucosa. **Tubular glands** with cells specialized for water absorption and **mucus-secreting goblet cells** are arranged closely packed together.

Answers

34. 1 – D, 2 – C, 3 – A, 4 – E, 5 – B
35. 1 – F, 2 – B, 3 – E, 4 – G, 5 – A, 6 – D, 7 – C

36. True or false? The stomach

A. Is where chyme formation takes place
B. Pylorus controls food entry to the stomach
C. Mucosa is thrown into folds called haustra
D. Has gastric pits which secrete gastric juice
E. Secretes gastrin from the pylorus

37. Regarding the stomach, which of the following statements are true?

a. It can hold up to 7 L of food
b. The fundus contacts the diaphragm
c. The cardiac sphincter is thickened by circular smooth muscle
d. Its blood supply is derived from the coeliac trunk
e. The stomach bed includes the pancreas

38. Consider the diagram of the stomach

a. What is indicated by the angular notch?
b. Label the diagram of the stomach using the following

Options

A. Body
B. Lesser curvature
C. Cardia
D. Oesophagus

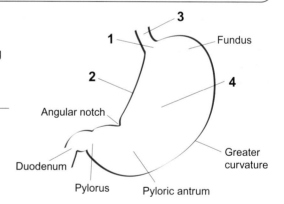

39. Concerning the blood supply to the stomach

a. Three branches of the coeliac trunk supply the stomach
b. The left gastric artery supplies the greater curvature
c. The short gastric arteries branch from the splenic artery
d. The left gastroepiploic artery lies between the layers of the gastrosplenic ligament
e. The left gastric artery has an oesophageal branch

APUD, amine precursor uptake and decarboxylation

EXPLANATION: PHYSIOLOGY OF THE STOMACH

The adult stomach can hold 2–3 L of food. It is fixed in place by two sphincters: the **cardiac sphincter**, which is strengthened by the diaphragm curling around it to prevent regurgitation, and the **pyloric sphincter**, which has circular smooth muscle to control flow of contents into the duodenum. The stomach bed upon which it lies, consists of **retroperitoneal** structures: the pancreas, left kidney, suprarenal gland, transverse colon and the spleen.

The mucosa of the stomach has three histologically different zones:

1. THE CARDIA   Contains mostly mucus-secreting glands. They surround the entrance of the oesophagus.

2. THE FUNDUS AND BODY   Contain gastric glands that consist of mucus-secreting mucus neck cells, parietal cells which secrete acid, chief cells which secrete pepsinogen (a precursor of pepsin) and APUD cells. The mucosa of the stomach is thrown into folds known as **rugae** which contain the gastric glands. They extend from the muscularis mucosae to open into the stomach lumen via gastric pits.

3. THE PYLORUS   Glands secrete mucus of two different types and have endocrine cells (G-cells) which secrete the hormone gastrin.

The angular notch is two-thirds along the lesser curvature and marks the junction between the body of the stomach and the pyloric part **(38b)**. The left gastric artery arises from the coeliac trunk. The right gastric artery arises from the hepatic artery. The right gastroepiploic artery arises from the terminal branches of the gastroduodenal artery. The left gastroepiploic artery arises from the splenic artery. Short gastric arteries arise from the splenic artery.

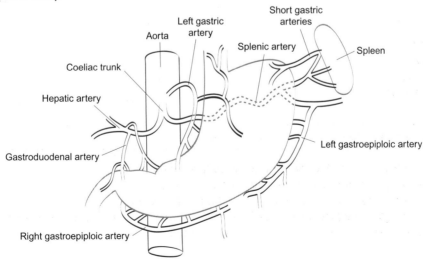

Answers
36. T F F F T
37. F T F T T
38a. See explanation
38b. 1 – C, 2 – B, 3 – D, 4 – A
39. T F T T T

40. True or false? Barrett's oesophagus

a. Occurs because of acid reflux
b. Is the metaplastic transformation of columnar epithelium
c. Is more common in smokers
d. Should be monitored regularly
e. Increases the risk of squamous cell carcinoma

41. Regarding cancer of the stomach

a. Gastric adenocarcinoma is more common in women than men
b. Ingestion of smoked foods is a risk factor
c. Gastric adenomatous polyps predispose to adenocarcinoma
d. There are three different patterns of growth of the tumour
e. It presents very early

42. Gastric carcinoma

a. May follow gastritis
b. Is more common in those with blood group O
c. Is most likely to be an adenocarcinoma
d. May spread to supraclavicular lymph nodes
e. Is associated with increased gastric acid secretion

43. The following are risk factors for chronic gastritis. True or false?

a. *Helicobacter pylori* infection
b. Heavy consumption of alcohol
c. Trauma
d. Aspirin ingestion
e. Vegetarianism

NSAID, non-steroidal anti-inflammatory drug

EXPLANATION: DISORDERS OF THE OESOPHAGUS AND STOMACH

Acid reflux oesophagitis may cause any of the following:

- Peptic ulceration
- Barrett's oesophagus
- Lower oesophageal stricture.

In **Barrett's oesophagus** squamous epithelium of the lower oesophagus is replaced by glandular epithelium composed of tall columnar cells (metaplasia). Patients should be kept under surveillance through endoscopy and biopsy to detect early neoplastic changes. Barrett's oesophagus puts the patient at risk of **adenocarcinoma**.

Gastritis is caused by inflammatory changes in the gastric mucosa and submucosa. It may be chronic or acute. Chronic gastritis may be ***Helicobacter pylori*** associated, autoimmune associated with pernicious anaemia, or reflux gastritis usually resulting from surgery to the pyloric region. This type of gastritis is also seen with prolonged NSAID use.

Complications of chronic gastritis include peptic ulceration and intestinal metaplasia, which may progress to carcinoma.

Gastric adenocarcinoma is more common in men and is associated with blood group A and the ingestion of smoked/salted preserved foods, due to the generation of nitrosamines by gut bacteria. People with **adenomatous polyps** are particularly at risk because of **malignant transformation**, as are those with gastritis.

Answers
40. T F T T F
41. F T T T F
42. T F T T F
43. T T F T F

44. Regarding the enteric nervous system

a. Vasoactive intestinal polypeptide relaxes sphincters
b. The myenteric plexus lies in the submucosa
c. Meissner's plexus lies between longitudinal and circular muscle
d. Stretch in the gut wall is sensed by neurons containing calcitonin-gene related polypeptide
e. Plexuses are isolated from each other

45. Concerning GI smooth muscle

a. The basic electrical rhythm is set at three contractions per minute
b. The pacemaker lies on the lesser curvature
c. Smooth muscle is arranged in bundles
d. Most gastrointestinal smooth muscle undergoes tonic contraction
e. Slow waves are associated with Ca^{2+} entry into the smooth muscle cells

GI, gastrointestinal; ACh, acetylcholine

EXPLANATION: GUT MOTILITY

GI motility is important to **move** food, **mix** it and bring it into **contact** with absorptive cells. It is controlled by both the extrinsic (**autonomic**) and intrinsic (**enteric**) nervous systems.

The smooth muscle of the gut is **myogenic**, that is it has its **own spontaneous electrical activity**. The **pacemaker** region is on the greater curvature of the stomach. It sets the basic electrical rhythm at three waves per minute. Impulses travel to the lesser curvature and the pyloric region. There are two types of electrical activity:

1. **Slow waves** are started in the pacemaker. They are oscillations within the resting membrane potential.
2. **Spike waves** occur at peaks of slow waves when membrane potential reaches a threshold of −40 mV.

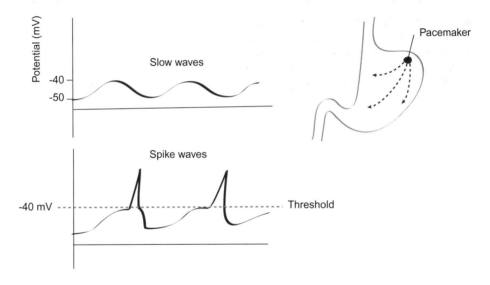

Both types of wave cause Ca^{2+} entry into the smooth muscle cells and therefore both types cause contraction. However the type of wave determines the type of contraction. Most GI smooth muscle contracts and relaxes in phases (phasic contraction) associated with slow waves and spikes. However sphincters undergo continuous (tonic) contraction, as a result of high frequency spike potentials.

The **enteric nervous system** consists of two networks of fibres: the myenteric (Auerbach's) plexus and the submucous (Meissner's plexus). They are interconnected within the GI tract. They contain **secretory**, **motor** and **sensory** neurons. They secrete many neurotransmitters, most importantly ACh and noradrenaline. Peristaltic activity is a result of the integrated function of the enteric system to sense the presence of food in the gut, and contract and relax the appropriate muscle. Peristalsis generally gets stronger towards the antrum, so that gastric contents are pressed towards the pylorus.

Answers
44. T F T T F
45. T F T F T

46. The following factors either (1) increase gastric motility, (2) decrease gastric motility, or (3) do not affect gastric motility. Group them accordingly

    A. Duodenal distension
    B. Histamine
    C. Gastrin
    D. Parasympathetic nerve supply
    E. Secretin

47. Concerning gastric motility, which of the following statements are true?

    a. When food is swallowed the cardiac sphincter contracts
    b. When food is swallowed the proximal stomach relaxes
    c. Peristalsis is particularly strong in the antrum
    d. Gastrin increases the frequency of the pacemaker
    e. The pacemaker produces oscillations every 20 seconds

CCK, cholecystokinin

EXPLANATION: CONTROL OF GUT MOTILITY

- When food reaches the stomach, there is receptive relaxation of the lower oesophageal sphincter by the **vagus** nerve.
- Peristalsis is a **reflex response** controlled by the enteric nervous system but it may be increased or decreased by the autonomic nervous system.
- **Parasympathetic cholinergic** activity increases muscle contractions; sympathetic noradrenergic activity decreases contractions but does contract the sphincters.
- Distension of the duodenum by chyme causes a vagal reflex (**iliogastric reflex**), which controls the rate at which it receives the chyme from the stomach.
- **Gastrin** is released from G-cells in the stomach in response to changes in the gastric contents. Not only does it stimulate gastric acid and pepsin secretion, it also increases gastric motility.
- **CCK** is secreted in response to intestinal amino acids, it inhibits gastrin release and therefore inhibits gastric emptying. It also augments the action of secretin, and stimulates satiety.
- **Secretin** causes the contraction of the pyloric sphincter, reduces gastric motility, inhibits gastric secretion and stimulates pancreatic secretion.

Answers
46. 1 – C, D; 2 – A, E; 3 – B
47. F T T T T

SECTION 2

LOWER GASTROINTESTINAL TRACT

2 LOWER GASTROINTESTINAL TRACT

---

1. Concerning the muscles of the anterior abdominal wall

a. The rectus abdominis originates from the pubic symphysis and the pubic crest
b. Fibres of the external oblique run upwards and forwards
c. The rectus sheath is formed by the aponeurosis of three anterior wall muscles
d. The nerve supply to the wall is exclusively from the lower six intercostal nerves
e. The erector spinae muscles contract to allow you to sit up in bed

---

2. The rectus abdominis muscle

a. Flexes the trunk
b. Is covered anteriorly by the aponeurosis of the external oblique and internal oblique
c. Is divided into four smaller muscle segments
d. Has an arcuate line indicating where it is not covered by the sheath posteriorly
e. Is separated in the midline by the linea semilunaris

---

3. Concerning the posterior abdominal wall

a. The iliopsoas is a flexor of the trunk and an extensor of the thigh
b. Psoas major inserts in the greater trochanter of the femur
c. Quadratus lumborum lies lateral to psoas major
d. The lumbar plexus is composed of L1–L3
e. The most superior nerve running across the wall is the subcostal nerve

EXPLANATION: MUSCLES OF THE ABDOMINAL WALL

The **external oblique muscle** is most superficial. The aponeuroses of this muscle, the **internal oblique muscle** and the innermost **transversus abdominis**, form the **rectus sheath** which encloses the **rectus abdominis** – a long muscle which lies on either side of the midline. External oblique fibres run downwards and forwards; internal oblique fibres run upwards and outwards.

The rectus abdominis is a broad strap-like muscle extending from the pubic symphysis and the pubic crest, attaching to the xiphoid process and the 5th–7th costal cartilages. It flexes the trunk and thoracoabdominal viscera. The muscle is enclosed by the rectus sheath which also contains superior and inferior epigastric arteries and veins, lymphatic vessels and ventral primary rami of T7–T12 nerves.

The posterior abdominal wall is made up from **psoas major**, **iliacus** and **quadratus lumborum**. The fibres of the iliacus join the tendon of psoas. Together they form the chief flexor of the thigh. The ventral rami of L1–L4 form the lumbar plexus which is in the posterior part of psoas major. The three largest branches of the plexus are the obturator nerve, the femoral nerve and the lumbrosacral trunk.

	Origin	Insertion
Muscles of anterior abdominal wall		
External oblique	External surfaces of 5th–12th ribs	Linea alba, pubic tubercle, anterior half of iliac crest
Internal oblique	Thoracolumbar fascia, anterior two-thirds of iliac crest, lateral half of inguinal ligament	Inferior borders of 10th–12th ribs, linea alba, conjoint tendon
Transverse abdominal	Internal surfaces of 7th–12th costal cartilages, thoracolumbar fascia, lateral third of inguinal ligament	Linea alba with aponeurosis of internal oblique, pubic crest, conjoint tendon
Rectus abdominis	Pubic symphysis and pubic crest	Xiphoid process, 5th–7th costal cartilages
Muscles of posterior abdominal wall		
Psoas major	Transverse processes of lumbar vertebrae, bodies of T12–L5 vertebrae	Lesser trochanter of femur
Iliacus	Superior two-thirds of iliac fossa, ala of sacrum and anterior sacroiliac ligaments	Lesser trochanter of femur and its shaft, psoas major tendon
Quadratus lumborum	Medial half of inferior border of 12th rib and tips of lumbar transverse processes	Iliolumbar ligament, internal lip of iliac crest

Answers

1. T F T F F
2. T T T T F
3. F F T F T

4. True or false? The inguinal ligament

a. Extends from the anterior superior iliac spine to the pubic crest
b. Is formed by the in-roll of the transverses abdominis aponeurotic fibres
c. Forms the pectineal ligament at the pubic crest
d. Contains the spermatic cord
e. Marks the location of the deep ring

5. The inguinal canal

a. Is 4 cm long in adults
b. Anterior wall is formed by the aponeurosis of the external oblique
c. Has a deep ring which lies just medial to the inferior epigastric artery
d. Has a non-palpable superficial ring
e. Is a rare site of hernias in both sexes

6. The spermatic cord

a. Passes through the inguinal canal
b. Has an innermost covering derived from the cremaster muscle
c. Carries the genital branch of the genitofemoral nerve
d. Drains lymph from the testis to the inguinal nodes
e. Can develop a hydrocele from the remnants of processus vaginalis

EXPLANATION: THE INGUINAL REGION

The **inguinal region** is particularly important anatomically since it is an area of weakness in the abdominal wall where hernias are prone to occur, especially in men. The inguinal ligament extends from the **anterior superior iliac spine** to the **pubic tubercle**. It is formed by the in-roll of the aponeurotic fibres of the external oblique. It forms the floor of the **inguinal canal** together with the lacunar ligament. The inguinal canal contains the **spermatic cord** in males.

The spermatic cord is contained within three layers of fascia, derived from the anterior abdominal wall. They are the **internal spermatic fascia**, derived from the transversalis fascia, the cremasteric fascia (and muscle) from the fasica of the internal oblique muscle, and the **external spermatic fascia** derived from the external oblique aponeurosis. The spermatic cord contains:

- Three arteries – testicular artery, cremasteric artery, artery of ductus deferens
- Three nerves – genital branch of genitofemoral nerve, ilioinguinal nerve fibres on arteries and ductus deferens (sympathetic and parasympathetic)
- Three veins – testicular vein, cremasteric vein, pampiniform plexus
- As well as the vas deferens and the lymphatics

Lymph from the **testis** drains to the **para-aortic nodes**, whereas lymph from the **scrotum** drains to the **inguinal** nodes.

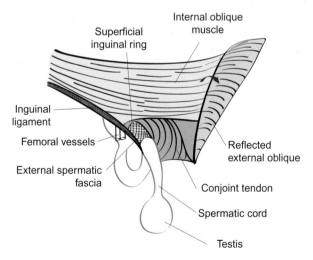

The inguinal canal is an oblique passage through the anterior abdominal wall. It has an opening at either end: the **deep and superficial rings**. The deep ring lies lateral to the **inferior epigastric artery**, its pulsations are a useful landmark to locate the ring.

Answers
4. F F F F F
5. T T F F F
6. T F T F T

7. Case study: inguinal hernia

A 52-year-old gardener comes into his GP's surgery one morning complaining of a lump in his groin. He claims he first noticed it about a week ago when he had been trying to repair the fence in his back garden. He felt a strange twinge as he lifted some planks of wood, but thought it was nothing until he noticed the lump, which he says sometimes disappears when he is lying down.

On examination, the lump was visible on the left side of the groin when the man stood. When he lay down the lump disappeared. The GP placed two fingers over the deep ring and asked the man to cough. When he removed his fingers the lump reappeared.

    a. What is meant by the term indirect inguinal hernia? How does this differ from direct hernia?

    b. How might this man be treated?

    c. What particular risks are involved with surgery to correct the hernia?

EXPLANATION: INGUINAL HERNIAS

Sixty per cent of groin hernias are **indirect inguinal**. They are most likely to result from failure of obliteration of the developmental processus vaginalis. The hernia protudes through the **deep ring** and along the **inguinal canal**. It may descend into the scrotum. Indirect hernias may be reduced (stroked back) to the deep ring and will not reappear unless you remove your finger from the deep ring, and raise intra-abdominal pressure (coughing, standing).

Direct hernias are less common, and are caused by protusion of the bowel through the posterior abdominal wall.

Uncomplicated hernias may be controlled using a truss (a pressure pad over the hernia) but it may be uncomfortable. Therefore, hernias may be repaired by open surgery or laparoscopic repair. In the case of indirect hernias the hernial sac is excised and the deep ring is tightened. Direct hernias can be invaginated back with sutures and reinforcement of the posterior wall of the inguinal canal.

Surgical excision endangers the **genitofemoral nerve** and **ilioinguinal nerve** (which provides cutaneous sensation to the top of the thigh, scrotum and penis). **Ductus deferens** may also be affected. Recurrence after surgery is common, usually due to incomplete excision of the sac. Also tightening the deep ring may **constrict the spermatic cord**.

Answers

7. See explanation

8. The duodenum

a. Is entirely retroperitoneal
b. Relates closely to the head of the pancreas
c. Lies posterior to the inferior vena cava
d. Receives the pancreatic duct and bile duct in its second part
e. Lies between L1 and L3

9. True or false? The jejunum

a. Has closer packed plicae circulares than the ileum
b. Mesentery contains less fat than the ileum
c. Is less vascular than the ileum
d. Has more complex arterial arcades than the ileum
e. Derives its blood supply from the superior mesenteric artery

10. Regarding the large intestine

a. The longitudinal muscular coat consists of taeniae coli
b. The caecum is retroperitoneal
c. The transverse colon is mostly supplied by the inferior mesenteric artery
d. The inner wall of the colon contains Peyer's patches
e. Its length can vary between 1.5 and 3.0 m

EXPLANATION: THE ANATOMY OF SMALL AND LARGE INTESTINES

The small intestine connects the colon to the stomach. The duodenum is essentially the beginning of the small intestine. It has **four parts**: superior, descending, horizontal and ascending. It is mostly retroperitoneal except for the very first 2.5 cm. This part is mobile, and is known as the **ampulla**. The inferior vena cava, the aorta and the right gonadal vein and artery lie behind the duodenum. Its blood supply is derived from the **superior mesenteric artery** (proximally) and the **coeliac trunk** (distally).

The jejunum joins the duodenum at the **duodenojejunal junction**. It mostly lies in the left upper quadrant of the abdomen. It is joined to the ileum – together they form 6–7 m of the small intestine. They each have distinctive characteristics, which are described in the table below. The **mesentery** is a fan of peritoneum that attaches the jejunum and ileum to the **posterior abdominal wall**.

	Jejunum	Ileum
Calibre	3.0 cm	1.5 cm
Length	~2.8 m	~4.2 m
Vascularity	Greater	Less
Mucosa	Circumferentially folded – plicae circulares	Randomly folded
Mesentery	Fewer arcades, large fenestrations	More arcades, small fenestrations
	Little fat	More fat
Lymphoid nodules	–	Peyer's patches

The large intestine begins at the ileocaecal junction. Indeed, it consists of the **caecum**, **appendix**, and the **ascending, transverse** and **descending colon**.

The caecum is a large dilated sac at the proximal end of the large intestine which lies in the right iliac fossa. The ileum opens into the caecum at the **ileocaecal valve**. The large intestine is supplied by both the foregut and midgut blood supplies. The distal third of the transverse colon onwards is supplied by the inferior mesenteric artery.

Answers
8. F T F T T
9. T T F F T
10. T T F F T

11. The large intestine can be distinguished from the small intestine by

a. The presence of taeniae coli
b. The fact that it is more vascular
c. Sacculations called haustra
d. Its larger internal diameter
e. Appendices epiploicae

12. Consider the cross-section of the colon below

a. Label the diagram of the ascending colon appropriately, where indicated
b. What is the origin of the artery supplying this part of the gastrointestinal tract?
c. Describe one way in which the large intestine can be distinguished anatomically from the small intestine

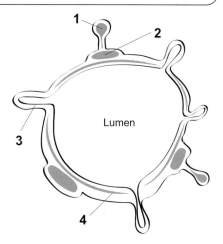

13. Regarding the GI tract

a. Label the parts indicated on the diagram opposite
b. What is the function of (1)?
c. What is the blood supply of (2)?

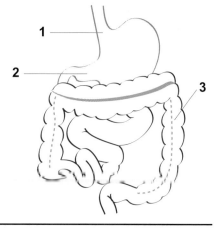

GI, gastrointestinal

EXPLANATION: THE COLON

Taeniae coli are three flat bands that form the circular muscular coat of the large intestine. Because taeniae are shorter than the intestine, the intestine is bunched up (sacculated) into **haustra**. There are no taeniae in the appendix or rectum. **Appendices epiploicae** are small sacs of fat that hang off the large intestine.

The oesophagus passes through the diaphragm at the level of **T10**, where it meets the stomach at the cardiac sphincter.

The cardiac and pyloric sphincters control the transit of food through the stomach. The pyloric sphincter is thickened by smooth circular muscle, and the cardiac sphincter is supported by the right crus of the diaphragm.

The developing GI tract is divided into foregut, midgut and hindgut, and the blood supplies of its components are based on these divisions.

- Foregut: coeliac trunk
- Midgut: superior mesenteric artery
- Hindgut: inferior mesenteric artery.

The first part of the duodenum lies at the level of L1. It is continuous with the stomach at the pylorus and is part of the foregut.

The rest of the duodenum is **retroperitoneal** and is part of the midgut, therefore it derives its blood supply from both the **coeliac trunk** (superior pancreaticoduodenal artery) and the **superior mesenteric artery** (inferior pancreaticoduodenal artery).

The blood supply for most of the colon comes from the superior mesenteric artery (right and middle colic branches) **(12b)**. However the distal third and the descending colon are supplied by the **left colic artery**, a branch of the inferior mesenteric artery. The inferior mesenteric artery continues inferiorly as the **superior rectal artery**.

Answers
11. T F T T T
12a. 1. Appendices epiploicae; 2. Taeniae coli; 3. Diverticulum; 4. Circular muscle; **12b.** See explanation; **12c.** See explanation
13a. 1. Cardiac sphincter; 2. Pyloric sphincter; 3. Descending colon; **13b.** To prevent regurgitation of food back up the oesophagus;
13c. Inferior mesenteric artery

14. True or false? The abdominal aorta

a. Enters the abdomen at T12
b. Bifurcates at L3
c. Bifurcates into the external and internal iliac arteries
d. Supplies the gut via three unpaired branches
e. Supplies the diaphragm via the superior phrenic arteries

15. The spleen

a. Is located in the right upper quadrant
b. Contacts the posterior wall of the stomach
c. Is retroperitoneal
d. Is supplied by the largest branch of the coeliac trunk
e. Is unlikely to be removed in the event of rupture

16. Regarding the appendix

a. It arises superior to the ileocaecal junction
b. It has a mesentery
c. It is supplied by a branch of the ileocolic artery
d. It is demarcated by McBurney's point
e. It is in the same position in everyone

EXPLANATION: THE SPLEEN AND APPENDIX

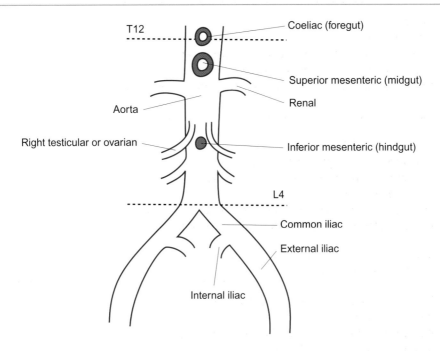

The **spleen** is the largest lymphatic organ. It is located in the left upper abdominal quadrant, and is completely covered in **peritoneum** except for the hilum. The relations of the spleen are: anteriorly, the posterior wall of the stomach, posteriorly, the left part of the diaphragm, inferiorly, the left colic flexure and medially, the left kidney. It is supplied by the splenic artery. The spleen may **rupture** on left-sided fracture to the 9th to 12th ribs, or because of a sudden increase in intra-abdominal pressure. In this case, repair of the spleen is very difficult so a **splenectomy** (removal) is usually performed.

The **vermiform appendix** is a blind-ended pouch of intestinal diverticulum that arises just below the ileocaecal junction. It has a short mesentery – mesoappendix – by which it is attached to the caecum. The caecum is supplied by the ileocaecal artery, a branch of the superior mesenteric artery. The appendix also derives its blood supply from the **ileocaecal artery**. Usually the appendix is **retrocaecal** and extends up towards the right colic flexure, however its position is variable between individuals. It may project towards the pelvis may even be fused to the abdominal wall.

McBurney's point is one-third of the way along a line joining the right anterior superior iliac spine to the umbilicus. The base of the appendix lies deep to this point.

Answers
14. T F F T F
15. F T F T F
16. F T T T F

17. The following are derivatives of the midgut

   a. Oesophagus
   b. Rectum
   c. Jejunum
   d. Descending colon
   e. Appendix

18. Regarding the development of the duodenum

   a. It rotates with the stomach to the right
   b. It lies externally to the peritoneum
   c. It becomes partially occluded in the fifth and sixth weeks' gestation
   d. It has three different blood supplies
   e. It is normally recanalized at birth

EXPLANATION: DEVELOPMENT OF THE MIDGUT (i)

Derivatives of the midgut include: the **small intestine** (including much of the duodenum distal to the duodenal papilla), the **caecum** and appendix, the **ascending colon**, and most of the **transverse colon** (except the distal third). The blood supply to the midgut is the **superior mesenteric artery**.

The duodenum epithelium arises from the caudal part of the foregut and the caudal part of the midgut. Other parts of the duodenum arise from surrounding mesenchyme. The duodenum rotates to gain its characteristic C-shaped loop, and becomes occluded in weeks 5 and 6 due to the proliferation of the epithelial lining cells. The lumen is usually recanalized in the eighth week. Failure of recanalization results in **duodenal stenosis**/atresia.

The entire midgut is suspended from the abdominal wall by an elongated dorsal (posterior) mesentery and communicates with the yolk sac through the yolk stalk. As it lengthens, the midgut forms a ventral U-shaped loop called **the midgut loop**. This projects into the proximal part of the umbilical cord because the liver and primitive gut take up space in the abdominal cavity. This projection is often referred to as the **midgut herniation (19a)**. It takes place during the sixth week of development. It remains in the umbilical cord until the end of the third month when it returns to the abdominal cavity (reduction).

The midgut herniation has cranial (headwards) and caudal (tailwards) parts: the cranial part lengthens rapidly to form loops of the small intestine whereas the caudal part undergoes very little change except for the development of a caecal bud, which later forms the caecum and appendix.

The midgut **rotates 90 degrees** anticlockwise around the superior mesenteric artery so that the cranial part is brought to the right and the caudal part is brought to the left. When reduction takes place, the intestines turn a further **180 degrees** anticlockwise, so that the cranial part (the small intestine) is now superior to the caudal part **(19b)**.

Answers
17. F F T F T
18. T T T F F

19. Answer the following questions on the midgut development

    a. What is meant by the term 'midgut herniation'?
    b. Describe briefly the rotation of the midgut
    c. What is Meckel's diverticulum?

20. Concerning the development of the anal canal

    a. The anal canal has a dual origin
    b. The cloacal membrane lies in the proctodeum
    c. The urogenital sinus divides the cloaca
    d. The ventral part of the cloaca develops into the anal canal
    e. The superior two-thirds of the anal canal is supplied by the superior rectal artery

EXPLANATION: DEVELOPMENT OF THE MIDUT (ii)

The final step in midgut development is **fixation** of the **intestines**. The mesentery attaching the intestines to the posterior abdominal wall is modified once reduction has taken place. The **mesentery** of the ascending and descending colon fuses with the parietal peritoneum on the posterior abdominal wall and disappears. As a result they both become retroperitoneal. The colon presses the duodenum against the posterior abdominal wall so that almost all of it becomes retroperitoneal.

Meckel's diverticulum (ileal diverticulum) is the most **common malformation** of the gut. It is a remnant of the proximal part of the yolk stalk that fails to degenerate during development, resulting in an outpouching of the ileum. It is usually 5 cm long, and projects 50 cm from the ileocaecal junction. Two per cent of the population have Meckel's diverticulum. It is usually symptomless but may cause rectal bleeding or abdominal pain.

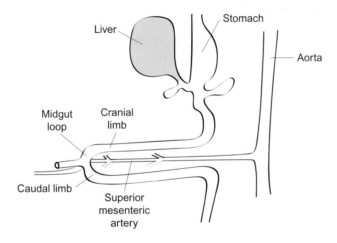

The caudal part of the hindgut is called the **cloaca**. This cavity contacts the ectoderm at the cloaca membrane, at the base of the proctodeum. The cloaca is divided into dorsal and ventral parts by the presence of the **urorectal septum**. The ventral portion is called the urogenital sinus, whereas the dorsal portion is called the anorectal canal. Where the urorectal septum fuses with the cloaca membrane is called the central **perineal tendon** or **perineal body**. The epithelium of the superior two-thirds of the anal canal arises from the hindgut, whereas the inferior third comes from the proctodeum. This dual origin is reflected in their differing blood supplies. The superior two-thirds is supplied by the superior rectal artery from inferior mesenteric artery, the inferior third is supplied by the inferior rectal arteries from the internal pudendal arteries.

Derivatives of the hindgut are: the distal third of the transverse colon, the descending colon, the sigmoid colon, rectum, superior part of the anal canal, and the epithelium of the urinary bladder and most of the urethra.

Answers
19. See explanation
20. T T F F T

21. With regard to the secretions of the small intestine

a. Alkaline mucus is secreted by the Brunner's gland
b. Bicarbonate ions are secreted in response to secretin
c. Enterocytes secrete water and electrolytes
d. Goblet cells secrete gastrointestinal hormones
e. The presence of chyme stimulates small intestine secretions

22. Fill in the gaps in the following paragraph about enzymatic aspects of digestion. Use the words from the list provided

Options

A. Pepsin
B. Brush border
C. Secretin
D. Stomach lumen
E. Oligopeptidase
F. Acidic
G. Co-lipase
H. Pancreas
I. Emulsion droplets
J. Alkaline
K. Salivary alpha amylase
L. Acid lipases
M. Cholecystokinin
N. Trypsin

Carbohydrate digestion begins in the oral cavity where starch is broken down by **1**. Fats and proteins are not broken down until they reach the **2**. Here, amylase is inactivated by the **3** pH, whereas **4** and **5** are activated. The mechanical action of the antrum is important to form small **6** of triglycerides and fatty acids. Once chyme reaches the duodenum, **7** and **8** are released. The **9** pH of the duodenum allows fatty acids to stabilize as smaller emulsion droplets. Pro-enzymes from the **10** are activated by the **11** cascade. **12** is particularly important as it allows pancreatic lipase to act on emulsion droplets. Protein digestion is completed by **13** on the small intestine **14**.

23. Concerning digestion in the small intestine, the following enzymes are present in the lumen of the duodenum

a. Alpha-amylase
b. Pepsin
c. Lipase
d. 11-beta Hydroxylase
e. Esterase

EXPLANATION: FUNCTION OF THE SMALL INTESTINE

The small intestine is responsible for digestion and absorption of end-products. On the surface of the small intestine mucosa are small pits called **crypts of Lieberkühn**, lying between the **intestinal villi**. They, like the villi, are covered by an epithelium composed of **goblet cells**, which secrete mucus, and enterocytes, which secrete water and electrolytes. Around 1.8 L of intestinal fluid is secreted per day, predominantly by the enterocytes. The secretions have a slightly alkaline pH. It should be noted that the watery secretion is reabsorbed again by the villi – thus it serves purely as a vehicle in which the products of digestion can be transported from the chyme to the intestinal mucosal cells. The mucosa of the small intestine also contains solitary and aggregated lymph nodules. Small glands in the duodenum called **Brunner's glands** secrete alkaline mucus to protect the duodenal mucosa from gastric acid.

Pancreatic secretions induced by the GI hormone secretin contain **bicarbonate ions**. Cl^- is secreted into the lumen via Cl^- channels activated by cAMP. The digestive enzymes in the duodenum lumen are those secreted from the pancreas (see page 107).

DIGESTION   Starch is broken down by both **salivary** and **pancreatic amylases**, which break alpha 1–4 linkages between glucose residues. They do not act on 1–6 branch linkages. The disaccharides produced are broken down in the small intestine lumen into monosaccharides by **brush border enzymes** such as sucrase, maltase and lactase.

Fat digestion begins in the stomach lumen. **Gastric lipase** is produced in the fundus, and begins hydrolysis of triglycerides. In the duodenum, bile secretion causes micelle/emulsion droplet formation which increases the surface area for pancreatic lipases to act. They are secreted in pro-form, to be activated by **trypsin**. **Co-lipase** displaces bile acids from emulsion droplets to allow lipase access to the triglycerides, which are broken down to free fatty acids and glycerol.

Protein digestion also begins in the stomach lumen. **Pepsin** attacks peptide bonds at a low pH to release a few amino acids and some smaller fragments of peptides. Once in the duodenum, **endopeptidases** activated by trypsin continue the hydrolysis, assisted by brush border enzymes specific to certain amino acids.

Answers
21. T T T F T
22. 1 – K, 2 – D, 3 – F, 4 – L, 5 – A, 6 – I, 7 – C, 8 – M, 9 – J, 10 – H, 11 – N, 12 – G, 13 – E, 14 – B
23. T F T F T

24. Draw a diagram of a villus. Label the following on your diagram

    A. Crypt of Lieberkühn
    B. Lacteal
    C. Microvilli
    D. Muscularis mucosa

25. Regarding absorption in the intestine

    a. Ninety per cent of Na^+ absorption takes place in the small intestine
    b. K^+ is absorbed by active transport
    c. Galactose and glucose compete for a co-transport carrier
    d. Amino acid absorption is increased by the presence of Na^+ in the lumen
    e. Free fatty acids are absorbed in the terminal ileum

ATP, adenosine triphosphate; ECF, extracellular fluid

EXPLANATION: ABSORPTION IN THE SMALL INTESTINE

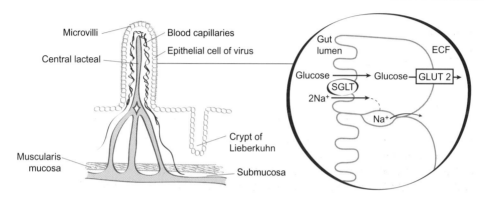

The absorptive surface of the small intestine is vastly increased in area by the **valvulae conniventes** (folds of mucosa), **villi** (covering the mucosa) and **microvilli** (covering the villi). Villi are finger-like projections which each contain a network of capillaries and a central lymphatic vessel called a **lacteal**. The epithelium of the villi are further divided into microvilli which form the **brush border** which contains many of the important enzymes of digestion.

ION ABSORPTION   The enterocytes are permeable to Na^+ so it can enter the mucosa by diffusion. Their basolateral membranes have **Na^+/K^+ ATPase** pumps to maintain a favourable concentration gradient to absorption. Na^+ is also actively reabsorbed. Cl^- ions tend to be dragged into the cells along with Na^+. Water also follows by osmosis. Some Na^+ is absorbed in exchange for secretion of K^+ or hydrogen ions. **Hydrogen** ions secreted into the lumen combine with **bicarbonate** ions (from bile and pancreatic juice) to form **carbonic acid** (**HCO_3**). They then dissociate to form water and carbon dioxide. Carbon dioxide is then readily absorbed by diffusion.

NUTRIENT ABSORPTION

- **Carbohydrate** – absorption of simple sugars such as glucose, fructose and galactose depends on **specific transport mechanisms** (carrier proteins). Glucose transport depends on Na^+ concentration in the lumen because **glucose** and **Na^+** ions share the same transporter (symport). The Na^+ gradient required for the functioning of this transport system is maintained by the basolateral Na^+/K^+ ATPase pump. This is therefore an active process (it requires ATP). Hexoses and pentoses are rapidly absorbed by simple diffusion across the wall of the small intestine.
- **Protein** – L-amino acids are absorbed more rapidly than their D-isomers. D-Amino acids are absorbed almost entirely by passive diffusion whereas most L-amino acids are actively transported. Transport is conducted by a variety of carriers. It is thought that Na^+ and some amino acids are transported together in much the same way that glucose is.

Answers
24. See diagram
25. T T T T T

26. Theme – transport across the gut epithelium. Match the following nutrients to their correct mechanism of absorption

Options

A. Simple passive diffusion
B. Facilitated diffusion
C. Primary active transport
D. Secondary active transport

1. Glucose
2. Alcohol
3. Fructose
4. Galactose
5. D-amino acids
6. Na$^+$ ions
7. Free fatty acids

27. Explain the following terms in association with the small intestine

a. MALT
b. Peyer's patches

GI, gastrointestinal; MALT, mucosal-associated lymphoid tissue

EXPLANATION: ABSORPTION IN THE GUT

Absorption of amino acids is **rapid** in the duodenum and jejunum but **slower** in the ileum. **Basic, acidic** and **neutral** amino acids are transported by **different mechanisms**. A congenital defect in the mechanism for the transport of neutral amino acids causes Hartnup disease, whereas a defect in the transport of basic amino acids causes cystinuria.

Monoglycerides, cholesterol and **fatty acids** from micelles are absorbed by **passive diffusion**. Fatty acids containing more than 10–12 carbon atoms are esterified into **triglycerides** within the small intestine mucosal cells. They are then packaged into **chylomicrons** and enter the **lymphatics**. Short-chain fatty acids pass straight from the mucosal cells into the **portal vein**.

Water is absorbed entirely by diffusion along an **osmotic gradient**. It can be transported in both directions, in other words from chyme to plasma, or plasma to chyme. This means that the chyme ends up isosmotic with the plasma.

MALT stands for mucosal-associated lymphoid tissue. Lymphoid tissue is distributed throughout the GI tract, either **diffusely**, or in discrete **aggregations**, for example the tonsils. The function of MALT is similar to that of lymph nodes. **Peyer's patches** are aggregations of lymphoid tissue in the small intestine, within the **lamina propria**. They have germinal centres containing lymphocytes.

Answers

26. 1 – D, 2 – A, 3 – B, 4 – D, 5 – A, 6 – C, 7 – A
27. See explanation

28. Divide the following causes of malabsorption into three groups: (1) very common, (2) uncommon, (3) rare

    A. Coeliac disease
    B. Chronic pancreatitis
    C. Whipple's disease
    D. Crohn's disease
    E. Resection of the stomach

29. The following are features of malabsorption. True or false?

    a. Frothy greasy pale stools
    b. Vomiting
    c. Diarrhoea
    d. Pernicious anaemia
    e. Bleeding disorders

30. Coeliac disease

    a. Is an abnormal reaction to starch
    b. Is characterized by villous atrophy
    c. Results in reduced gastrointestinal hormone secretion
    d. Improves the prognosis for small bowel cancer
    e. Is treated by cutting out carbohydrate

EXPLANATION: DISORDERS OF ABSORPTION

Malabsorption in the small intestine occurs as a result of impairment of one of the following factors:

- Secretion of **pancreatic hydrolytic enzymes**
- Secretion of **bile**
- Functional **villi** in the absorptive mucosa
- **Brush border enzymes**.

Thus, **pancreatic insufficiency** is a common cause of malabsorption. Examples include **cystic fibrosis**, **chronic pancreatitis**, **cancer** of the pancreas and pancreatic **surgery**. **Coeliac disease** is the most important cause of malabsorption in industrialized countries.

Causes of malabsorption reducing the absorptive surface area of the mucosa include Crohn's disease, infarction and resection of the small bowel.

The effects of malabsorption are:

- Pale frothy stools which float because of their high fat and gas content (steatorrhea)
- Osmotic diarrhoea: water remains in the lumen because of the inadequate absorption of osmotic particles (nutrients)
- Weight loss
- Anaemia due to the deficiency in iron, folate or vitamin B12 caused by malabsorption
- Bleeding disorders due to poor absorption of vitamin K (clotting factor)
- Oedema resulting from low protein.

Coeliac disease is caused by an abnormal reaction to **gluten** found in **wheat**, **rye**, **barley** and **oats**. It causes an enteropathy in the **jejunal mucosa** characterized by a **loss of villous** architecture and **deepening of crypts**. The toxic element is the protein **gliadin**, a component of gluten. It induces a lymphocytic immune response. Withdrawal of gluten from the diet leads to a recovery of normal architecture which may be partial or complete. The condition may predispose to cancer of the small intestine.

Answers

28. 1 – A, B; 2 – D, E; 3 – C
29. T F T T T
30. F T T F F

31. Match the following bacteria to the part of the alimentary tract where they are commonly found

Options

A. Oropharynx
B. Stomach
C. Small intestine
D. Large intestine

1. *Streptococcus viridans*
2. *Enterococcus faecalis*
3. *Clostridia*
4. *Helicobacter pylori*
5. *Lactobacillus*
6. *Escherichia coli*

32. Concerning the flora of the intestinal tract

a. The colon is sterile at birth
b. Bacteria in the colon are predominantly aerobic
c. Bacteria convert conjugated bilirubin to urobilinogen
d. Bacteria convert fatty acids to simple sugars
e. Bacteria deconjugate sex hormones

33. Regarding antibiotic therapy

a. What type of antibiotic therapy is necessary when considering large bowel surgery?
b. Why might someone taking broad-spectrum antibiotics develop diarrhoea?

EXPLANATION: FLORA OF THE GUT

The normal healthy human body has a whole array of **commensal bacteria** which exist symbiotically with their host. This is known as the flora of the human body. These bacteria are harmless and may even be beneficial in some cases.

In the gut, bacteria maintain the normal structure and function of the intestine. They **degrade mucins**, **epithelial cells** and **fibre**, and they produce certain **vitamins**. They also convert conjugated bilirubin to urobilinogen and stercobilinogen, and convert disaccharides to short-chain fatty acids. Commensal bacteria usually help to prevent attack by pathogenic bacteria by competing for space and nutrients. However, commensal bacteria can become **pathogenic** if they gain access to sites they do not usually inhabit. For this reason it is vital to learn the normal distribution of flora. The main bacteria in the gut are listed below.

Site	Organisms
Oropharynx	*Streptococcus viridans*
	Neisseria
	Corynebacteria
	Bacteroides
Stomach	Usually sterile (*H. pylori*)
Small intestine	*Streptococcus*
	Lactobacillus
Colon	*Escherichia coli*
	Enterococci
	Bacteroides
	Proteus
	Klebsiella

The stomach is usually **sterile** due to the secretion of gastric acid, but it may be colonized by *Helicobacter pylori*. The flora of the small intestine is sparse, but the large intestine is very heavily colonized by anaerobic bacteria. The bacteria in the faeces make up a third of its weight!

Before surgery on the intestines, the aim is to attain a site as 'clean' as possible. Ideally **cefuroxime** is given to kill gram-negative coliforms and neisseria, and **metronidazole** is given to kill gram-negative and -positive anaerobes **(33a)**. Antibiotics are generally given parenterally.

Diarrhoea is a common side effect of broad-spectrum oral antibiotic therapy. It occurs because the suppression of normal commensal flora of the large intestine allows *Clostridium difficile* to overgrow **(33b)**. *C. difficile* is acquired from the environment or from other patients.

Answers
31. 1– D, 2 – D, 3 – B, 4 – C, 5 – D
32. T F T F T
33. See explanation

34. Concerning absorption in the colon

a. The colon can absorb a maximum of 5 L per day of fluid and electrolytes
b. Most of the absorption in the colon takes place in its proximal half
c. It is insensitive to aldosterone
d. Bicarbonate ions are absorbed in exchange for Cl^-
e. Paracellular spaces are important to the secretion of K^+

35. Diarrhoea

a. Is caused by a failure of water absorption in the intestines
b. Is never lethal
c. Causes a metabolic alkalosis
d. Can be caused by cholera toxin
e. May occur as a result of malabsorption of nutrients

ATP, adenosine triphosphate

EXPLANATION: ABSORPTION IN THE COLON

One and a half litres of chyme pass into the large intestine each day. Ninety per cent of the water is absorbed, leaving behind a small volume of faecal material which is mostly water. The mucosa of the large intestine has a high capability for **active absorption of Na⁺ ions** – wherever Na⁺ goes, **water** follows because of the osmotic gradient created across the mucosa. **Cl⁻ ions** also follow Na⁺. From the mucosal cell, Na⁺ and Cl⁻ are pumped into paracellular spaces, in exchange for **K⁺ ions**. K⁺ is then driven into the lumen of the intestine because of the electronegative potential in the lumen.

Tight junctions between the cells prevent back diffusion of Na⁺ ions and **aldosterone** increases Na⁺ transport. The large intestine also secretes **bicarbonate** ions in exchange for the absorption of Cl⁻ ions. Bicarbonate helps to neutralize the contents of the lumen.

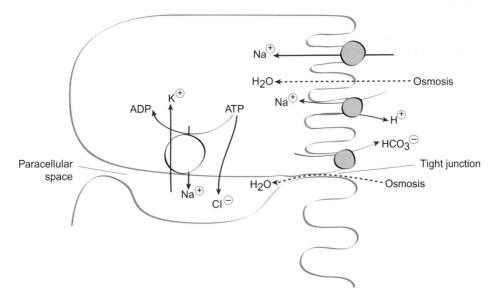

Diarrhoea may be osmotic, secretory, exudative or due to deranged motility. Basically, it occurs because the mechanism by which the water is **absorbed** from the colon is **impaired**.

Diarrhoea causes the loss of **water** and **bicarbonate ions** (remember they are secreted into the lumen of the intestine) from the body. The result is **dehydration** and a **metabolic acidosis** – a surplus of hydrogen ions. The person should take water and NaCl (i.e. oral rehydration solution) and allow the kidneys to restore the normal balance of ions by excreting HCl and retaining NaHCO₃.

Answers
34. T T F F T
35. T F F T T

36. Regarding laxative agents, which of the following statements are true?

a. Methylcellulose is a bulk laxative
b. They increase transit time through the colon
c. Lactulose has no side effects
d. Osmotic laxatives increase water content in the lumen
e. Magnesium hydroxide is a laxative

37. Constipation may be relieved by

a. Increasing the fibre content of the diet
b. Loperamide
c. Magnesium sulphate
d. Liquid paraffin
e. Stimulating the myenteric plexus

38. The following are important in the management of acute diarrhoea

a. Oral rehydration solution
b. Loperamide
c. Metoclopramide
d. Senna
e. Magnesium aluminium silicate

EXPLANATION: CONSTIPATION AND LAXATIVES

There are two types of laxative:

1. BULK LAXATIVES   act by increasing the volume of non-absorbable residue in the lumen of the intestine. Examples are methycellulose, bran, agar. They take a few days to work, their advantage being that they have no side effects, and are the most natural method of purging the colon.

2. OSMOTIC LAXATIVES   act by increasing the volume of fluid in the lumen of the intestine by osmosis. This reduces transit time through the small intestine, resulting in a large volume entering the large intestine, the result is purgation within an hour. Examples are salts of Mg^{2+}. They can cause abdominal cramps, diarrhoea and electrolyte disturbances. Lactulose is an osmotic laxative.

Fibre adds bulk to stool to increase the **mechanical efficiency** of the intestine, and **absorbs water** to soften the stool. Its deficiency is a very common cause of constipation in the elderly. Salts containing poorly absorbed ions make good osmotic laxatives. Loperamide is an opioid used as an antidiarrhoeal not a laxative because of its local effect.

Short episodes of diarrhoea are very common and often do not require clinical investigation or treatment. However, if severe, causing dehydration or associated with fever, vomiting and abdominal pain, diarrhoea may be a risk to the health of the vulnerable, particularly the old and the young.

Acute diarrhoea should be managed primarily with oral fluid and electrolyte replacement. Special **rehydration solutions** such as diarolyte can be given. Although antidiarrhoeals are generally disapproved of because they impair clearance of the pathogen, they can be given for short-term relief (e.g. **loperamide**). Adsorbent agents such as **charcoal**, **chalk** and **magnesium aluminium silicate** have not been proved to provide any benefit, but are thought to protect the intestinal mucosa.

Senna is a laxative and **metoclopramide** increases gut motility.

Answers
36. T F F T T
37. T F T T T
38. T T F F F

39. Regarding inflammatory bowel disease

a. Complete this table of differences between Crohn's disease and ulcerative colitis

	Crohn's disease	Ulcerative colitis
Location	1	Large intestine only, especially rectum
Inflammation	Granulomatous pattern Affects full thickness of bowel wall (transmural) Discontinuous (skip lesions)	3 Affects mucosa and lamina propria Continuous
Ulceration	2	Shallow ulceration, haemorrhagic
Malignancy	+ risk	4

b. List three systemic complications of ulcerative colitis

40. True or false? Diverticular disease

a. Affects a third of the population over 35 years old
b. Is seen most commonly in the transverse colon
c. Is associated with raised intraluminal pressure
d. May result in perforation
e. May cause intestinal obstruction

41. Concerning appendicitis

a. Pain is initially felt in the umbilical region
b. Pain can be relieved by applying pressure to McBurney's point
c. It may cause peritonitis
d. It only affects children
e. It is treated by appendectomy

42. Hirschsprung's disease

a. Is caused by an absence of parasympathetic efferents to the gut
b. Is associated with children with Down's syndrome
c. Is often associated with early life gastroenteritis
d. May cause intestinal obstruction
e. Is characterized by megacolon

EXPLANATION: BOWEL DISEASES

The two main chronic inflammatory bowel diseases are **Crohn's disease** and **ulcerative colitis**. Inflammatory bowel disease is generally more common in western countries. The cause is not known although there is a familial tendency. **Smoking increases** the risk of **Crohn's** but is protective against **ulcerative colitis**. Symptoms depend on the region of the bowel affected, however both diseases tend to present as relapses and remissions of **diarrhoea**, **bleeding**, **abdominal pain** and **weight loss**. Systemic manifestations include conjunctivitis (eyes), arthritis, ankylosing spondylitis (joints), erythema nodosum (skin), fatty change in the liver and chronic liver disease **(39b)**.

Diverticular disease (**diverticulosis**) is the herniation of the mucosa and submucosa through the circular muscle of the wall of the large intestine. It is rare under the age of 35 but affects a third of the population over 65 years old. Contributing factors are: **weakness** of the bowel wall, raised **intraluminal pressure**, an **age-related reduction** in the strength of colonic connective tissue, and a **low dietary fibre** intake. Symptoms only arise from complications, such as: inflammation resulting in diverticulitis, perforation of a pericolic abscess, fistula formation, intestinal obstruction and bleeding.

Inflammation of the appendix causes early pain in the **umbilical region** because afferent pain fibres from the appendix enter the spinal cord at T10. As the peritoneum overlying the appendix becomes inflamed, the pain spreads to the **right iliac fossa**. Flexion of the right thigh relieves the pain somewhat, as it causes relaxation of right psoas major.

Hirschsprung's disease affects 1 in 5000 babies. It is caused by the absence of ganglion cells from the **Auerbach's** and **Meissner's plexus** in the distal large bowel. It is normally associated with congenital abnormalities, particularly Down's syndrome.

Because the parasympathetic plexuses fail, peristalsis is lost and a segment of the bowel goes into spasm. This causes the intestine proximal to the segment to become distended with faeces and dilate (megacolon). Ischaemic enterocolitis may then develop, leading to death.

Answers

39a. 1. Anywhere in the alimentary tract, especially mouth, terminal ileum, colon, anus; 2. Deep ulcers and fissures, 'cobblestone appearance'; 3. No granulomas, goblet cell depletion, crypt abscesses; 4. +++ risk; **39b.** See explanation
40. F F T T T
41. T F T F T
42. F T F T T

43. Regarding the rectum and anal canal

a. The lower third of the rectum is entirely covered by peritoneum
b. The anal canal begins as the bowel passes though the pelvic floor
c. The pectinate line demarcates a change in blood supply
d. The internal anal sphincter is supplied by voluntary nerve fibres
e. The internal anal sphincter contracts on sympathetic stimulation

44. Consider the rectum and anal canal

a. Explain briefly the mechanism of defecation
b. Label the diagram of the rectum and anal canal below

Options

A. Rectum
B. Sigmoid colon
C. Levator ani

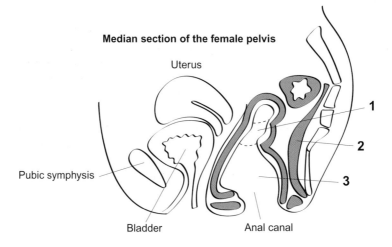

Median section of the female pelvis

Uterus

Pubic symphysis

Bladder

Anal canal

1

2

3

EXPLANATION: RECTUM AND ANUS

The sigmoid colon and rectum are continuous at the level of vertebrae S2/S3. The rectum follows the curve of the sacrum and the coccyx – forming the sacral flexure. The upper third of the rectum is covered with peritoneum on its anterior and lateral surfaces, whereas the middle third is covered with peritoneum anteriorly only. The inferior third is not covered at all. This is because the peritoneum is reflected forwards onto the bladder in the male or vagina in the female.

On either side of the rectum are the **levator ani** muscles, or the **pelvic diaphragm**. The rectum mucous membrane is thrown into transverse folds.

The **superior rectal artery** (from the inferior mesenteric artery) and the two middle rectal arteries supply the proximal part of the rectum up to the **pectinate line**. Below the pectinate line (immediately below the anal valves – remnants of the embryonic proctodeum membrane), the **inferior rectal arteries** (from the internal pudendal arteries) supply the anorectal junction and the anal canal.

The anal canal begins where the rectum pierces the pelvic diaphragm. It is about 2.5–3.5 cm long. The superior half of the anal canal has a mucous membrane characterized by folds called **anal columns**. The **anorectal junction** is where the superior ends of the anal columns join the rectum; the inferior ends of the anal columns form the **anal valves**.

The two sphincters controlling passage of faeces are concentric. The internal anal sphincter is **smooth muscle**. It is basically a thickening of circular and longitudinal muscle from the rectum. The internal sphincter is tonically contracted most of the time to prevent escape of faeces/fluid. It relaxes **involuntarily** in response to pressure from faeces distending the rectal ampulla **(44a)**. Part of the levator ani muscle, the pubo-rectalis forms a sling around the ano-rectal junction, which assists the internal sphincter in contraction.

Skeletal muscle from the levator ani forms the external anal sphincter. This is a **voluntary sphincter** which is supplied by the pudendal nerves (S4). It is voluntarily contracted to prevent defecation.

The anal canal ends at the anus – the external outlet of the GI tract.

Answers
43. F T T T T
44a. See explanation; **44b.** 1 – B, 2 – C, 3 – A

45. Case study: Haemorrhoids

A 32-year-old woman comes to see her GP one afternoon because she has noticed blood stains on the toilet paper after passing stool for the past 4 days. She is 26 six weeks pregnant and worried something might be wrong with her baby. On further questioning, she admits that she has noticed some mucus discharge in her stool.

    a. What are haemorrhoids? How are they classified?

    b. What are the risk factors for haemorrhoids?

    c. Why might this woman feel tired and lethargic?

    d. Is it possible her symptoms could be explained by any other pathology?

EXPLANATION: DEFECATION AND HAEMORRHOIDS

Mass movement of **faeces** from the **sigmoid colon** to the rectum **distends** this chamber and causes stretch receptors to send impulses via the **parasympathetic** afferents of sacral nerves **2, 3** and **4**. In children who have not yet been potty-trained, a reflex arc causes inhibition of the internal sphincter by sympathetic efferents from L1 and 2 so that it relaxes, and there is also relaxation of the external sphincter via the pudendal nerves (S3 and 4). Presynaptic parasympathetic outflow causes the smooth muscle of the rectal wall to contract, resulting in peristaltic waves to expel faeces. In older children and adults, **ascending pathways** from the spinal cord to the cerebral cortex make us **aware** of the need to defecate, and therefore descending pathways inhibit the reflex arc if inappropriate.

Haemorrhoids or piles, as they are more commonly known, are the commonest cause of rectal bleeding. The anus is lined by **three vascular cushions**, attached by smooth muscle and elastic tissue. They drain via the superior rectal veins into the inferior mesenteric vein. Gravity, increased anal tone and straining at stool all weaken the supporting framework of these cushions, so they become loose and protude. They are then vulnerable to trauma and bleeding. Risk factors are a **history of constipation, pregnancy, portal hypertension** and **rectal carcinoma (45b)**.

Haemorrhoids are classified as **primary, secondary** and **tertiary (45a)**. Primary piles remain in the rectum. Secondary piles prolapse through the anus on defecation but spontaneously reduce. Tertiary piles remain outside the anus at all times. **Bright red rectal bleeding,** mucus discharge, pruritus ani and anaemia are all features **(45c)**.

It is possible that in this case study the woman's symptoms are caused by a perianal haematoma, anal fissure or abscess, or even a tumour **(45d)**. Therefore further investigations are always required.

Answers

45. See explanation

HEPATOBILIARY SYSTEM AND PANCREAS

3

HEPATOBILIARY SYSTEM AND PANCREAS

1. The liver

a. Receives 25 per cent of its blood supply from the portal vein
b. Contains 50 000–100 000 lobes
c. Has its own specialized macrophages
d. Is composed of functional units called acini
e. Receives 29 per cent of the cardiac output

2. True or false? The liver

a. Is innervated by the coeliac plexus
b. Develops from endodermal epithelium
c. Is more susceptible to ischaemic damage in the perivenous area of the acini
d. Can store up to 3 L of extra blood
e. Can perform haematopoiesis

3. The liver performs the following functions

a. Ca^{2+} homeostasis
b. Formation of bile
c. Storage of vitamins
d. Gluconeogenesis
e. Insulin synthesis

EXPLANATION: THE LIVER – STRUCTURE AND FUNCTION

The **liver** is the largest gland in the body. It lies **beneath** the dome of the **diaphragm** and the central tendon on the **right side of the body**.

It is composed of **four lobes** – right, left, caudate and quadrate – which contain within them 50 000–100 000 lobules. A lobule can be thought of as a cylindrical structure of hepatic cells (**hepatocytes**) surrounding a **central vein**. However the liver is sometimes described as being arranged into **acini**, with the **portal triad** at the centre. This arrangement is used to emphasize the **endocrine function** of the liver.

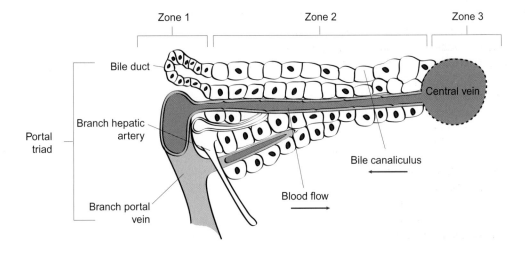

The **acini** are divided into **three zones** to reflect the metabolic gradient of the liver. The **centre** of the **acinus** (periportal area or zone 1) receives the most **oxygenated blood**. As blood filters peripherally, oxygen is used up. Zone 3 is the least oxygenated. However, zone 1 is most susceptible to damage from ingested toxins via the portal blood.

Innervation to the liver is by the **hepatic plexus**, a derivative of the **coeliac plexus**. The plexus contains branches from the **vagus** nerves and the **phrenic** nerves. The nerves contain both sympathetic and parasympathetic fibres.

The liver has numerous functions, principally to do with **metabolism. Glucose** and **glycogen** are both synthesized in the liver, **fatty acids** are synthesized and packaged into triglycerides for transport in lipoproteins. **Cholesterol** is also synthesized here. Important plasma proteins such as **albumin** and **clotting factors** are formed, and **amino acids** are deaminated for the formation of **urea**. The liver also produces **bile**, acts as a store for vitamin A, D and B12, and detoxifies drugs and foreign compounds.

Answers
1. F F T T T
2. T T T F T
3. F T T T F

4. Regarding the anatomical lobes of the liver

a. They are approximately equal in size
b. The caudate lobe lies between the fissure for ligamentum venosum and the fossa for the inferior vena cava
c. The falciform ligament divides the liver into functional left and right lobes
d. The bare area of the liver is in direct contact with the diaphragm
e. The gallbladder fossa lies in the quadrate lobe

5. Regarding the liver surface anatomy

a. The liver lies between ribs seven and eleven
b. The liver moves superiorly during inspiration
c. The inferior border follows the costal margin
d. The liver is located more inferiorly when erect
e. The liver is positioned such that it is not easily injured

6. Fill in the gaps in the following paragraph about the anatomy of the liver, using the words from the list below. You may use each word once, more than once, or not at all

Options

A. Diaphragm	B. Falciform ligament
C. Porta hepatis	D. Visceral
E. Left	F. Right upper quadrant
G. Bare area	H. Parietal
I. Portal vein	J. Hepatorenal recess
K. Quadrate	L. Subphrenic recesses

The liver lies mainly in the **1**, just below the inferior surface of the diaphragm. Much of the anterior and superior parts of the liver are tucked under the **2**, however, they are prevented from contacting it by the **3**. This diaphragmatic surface of the liver is entirely covered in **4** peritoneum except for the **5**, posteriorly; it begins where the peritoneum forms the coronary ligament. The visceral surface of the liver is also covered with peritoneum except at the **6**, a transverse fissure between caudate and **7** lobes which allows entry of the hepatic artery and **8**.

GB, gallbladder; IVC, inferior vena cava

EXPLANATION: THE LIVER – ANATOMY

Anterior view

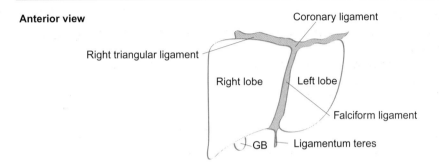

Visceral surface (posterior view)

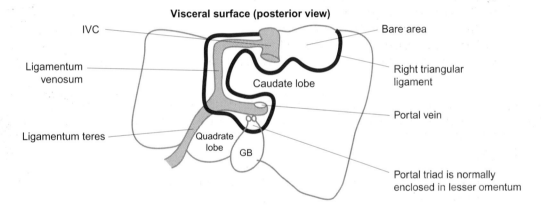

The **liver** lies between **ribs seven** and **eleven**, in the **right upper quadrant** of the abdomen. The lower border extends from the tip of the tenth rib to just below the left nipple. It may be **palpable** in a **normal subject**, particularly on inspiration, when it moves inferiorly.

Recognizing boundaries for the lobes of the liver can be tricky since there are functional definitions and, of course, anatomical definitions. The liver is divided into two equal sized **functional** lobes by an imaginary line running through the gallbladder fossa and inferior vena cava. However, the right and left **anatomical** lobes of the liver are demarcated based on the position of the lesser omentum (connecting liver to gut) and falciform ligamen (attaches liver to anterior abdominal wall). Both these mesenteries are derived from the anterior mesentery in the developing gut, which the liver grows into.

7. True or false? The space of Disse

a. Lies between the endothelial cells of sinusoids and hepatic cells
b. Connects with lymphatic vessels
c. Transports bile to bile canaliculi
d. Contains large plasma proteins
e. Consists of large pores in the endothelial lining

8. Bile canaliculi

a. Run intracellularly in hepatic cords
b. Are sealed by tight junctions
c. Form part of a portal triad
d. Empty into canals of Hering
e. May transport blood

9. The hepatic portal vein

a. Has a pressure of about 10 mmHg
b. Drains blood from the liver to the inferior vena cava
c. Has no vasodilatory innervation
d. Supplies the peripheral portion of the acinus better than the centre
e. Blood does not mix with the hepatic artery blood

10. The portal vein

a. Is formed by the union of the splenic vein and left gastric vein
b. Contains blood which is poorly oxygenated
c. Contains blood which is nutrient-rich
d. Drains the entire gastrointestinal tract
e. Communicates with the systemic circulation via anastamoses

EXPLANATION: LIVER MICROSTRUCTURE

Here we look in further detail at the microstructure of the liver. Networks of capillaries called **sinusoids** lie between hepatocytes in the liver. The endothelial cells are separated from the hepatic cells by a narrow tissue space called the **space of Disse**. Large pores in the endothelium allow plasma to move freely into the space. In the **fetus**, the space of Disse contains **haematopoietic cells**.

Bile canaliculi are small canals which lie between adjacent hepatic cells. They receive bile from hepatocytes, drain into **canals of Hering**, which then drain into bile ducts, which form part of the portal triad.

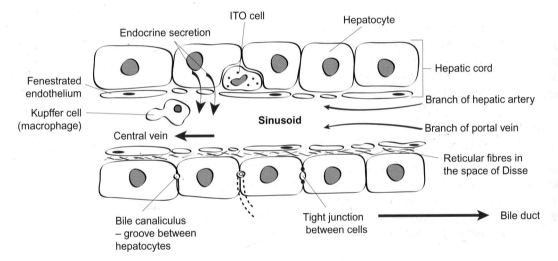

Branches of the **hepatic portal vein** form part of the **portal triad** together with the **hepatic artery** and **bile duct**. It transports solutes from the gut to the liver for metabolism. **Seventy-five per cent of the blood supply to the liver is from the hepatic artery** – the blood mixes in the sinusoids. The **hepatic portal vein** also delivers blood (at a rate of 1 L/min) to the liver. It is formed from the splenic, superior mesenteric and inferior mesenteric veins, in addition to other smaller tributaries just behind the neck of the pancreas. The portal vein terminates at the **porta hepatis** (a transverse fissure between caudate and quadrate lobes), where it divides into right and left branches. The portal venous system communicates with the systemic venous system via anastamoses at the oesophagus, the rectum, the anterior abdominal wall and the colon.

Answers

7. T T F T F
8. F T F T F
9. T F T F F
10. F T T T T

11. True or false? The following factors stimulate bile secretion by the liver

    a. Increased hepatic blood flow
    b. Contraction of the gallbladder
    c. Vagal stimulation
    d. Secretin
    e. Low concentration of bile acid in blood

12. Bile has the following functions

    a. To digest fat
    b. To bind amino acids and aid their transport across the intestinal mucosal membrane
    c. To neutralize acid chyme
    d. To emulsify fat particles
    e. To transport waste products away from the liver

13. Regarding bile acids

    a. Their synthesis is catalysed by cholesterol 7 alpha hydroxylase
    b. They are degraded in the terminal ileum
    c. A deficiency causes malabsorption of fat
    d. They are bound by resins to reduce hyperlipidaemia therapeutically
    e. They may be conjugated to form bilirubin

14. True or false? The bile duct

    a. Is formed by the union of the pancreatic duct and the cystic duct
    b. Varies from 5 to 15 cm in length
    c. Descends posterior to the first part of the duodenum
    d. Releases bile directly into the large intestine
    e. Opens in the wall of the gut at the ampulla of Vater

EXPLANATION: BILE SECRETION

Bile contains **water**, **bile acids**, **cholesterol**, **lipids** and the **bile pigments** bilirubin and biliverdin.

Around 500 mL of **bile** is **secreted** by the liver per day. It helps to **emulsify** large fat particles so that they can easily be attacked by the **lipase** enzyme secreted in the pancreatic juice. It also aids their transport through the intestinal mucosal membrane and removes waste products (including **bilirubin**) from the liver.

The main bile pigment, **bilirubin**, comes from the breakdown of **haemoglobin** in old red blood cells. This takes place in the reticuloendothelial system. Bilirubin is then transported to the liver by the circulation bound to albumin, since it is insoluble.

Bile acids are **synthesized** in the **hepatocytes** themselves. They are all formed from **cholesterol**. Bile salts are then formed from these acids by conjugation with K^+ or Na^+. Primary bile salts are formed in the liver. They are then modified by bacteria in the colon to form secondary bile salts.

The **hepatocytes** secrete these components in the form of bile into the small intestine where **90–95 per cent** of the bile salts/acids are **reabsorbed** (mostly in the terminal ileum) and enter the **portal vein** to be transported back to the liver for recycling. This is known as **enterohepatic recirculation**. For this reason we only synthesize a small amount of bile acids.

The bile pigments **bilirubin** and **biliverdin** are normally excreted in the **faeces**.

Factors that increase the secretion of bile by the liver are known as **choleterics**. They include stimulation by the vagus nerve, secretin and, most importantly, the bile salts themselves.

Answers
11. T F T T F
12. F F F T T
13. T F T T F
14. F T T F F

15. The gallbladder

a. Contracts in response to cholecystokinin
b. Holds a maximum of 500 mL of bile
c. Empties by contraction of the sphincter of Oddi
d. Is stimulated by the vagus nerve
e. Concentrates bile up to 15 times

16. With regard to the gallbladder

a. It lies in the cystic fossa of the liver
b. It has a capacity of up to 50 mL of bile
c. It is supplied by a branch of the splenic artery
d. It contacts the ascending colon
e. It receives a parasympathetic nerve supply from the vagus

17. Label the diagram below as indicated

Options

A. Pancreatic duct
B. Left hepatic duct
C. Fundus
D. Neck
E. Liver
F. Pancreas
G. Hepato-pancreatic ampulla
H. Bile duct
I. Common hepatic duct
J. Cystic duct

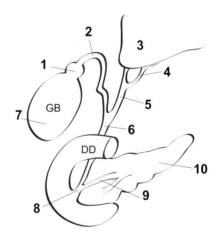

18. Concerning the gall bladder

a. What causes the gallbladder to contract?
b. How is the composition of bile changed in the gallbladder?
c. Name three factors that help the sphincter of Oddi to relax

CCK, cholecystokinin; DD, duodenum; GB, gallbladder

EXPLANATION: THE GALLBLADDER

The **gallbladder** has three parts, the **fundus**, **body** and **neck**. The fundus lies at the margin of the liver, and the body lies against the transverse colon, in front of the first part of the duodenum. It narrows into the neck from which the cystic duct opens. The gallbladder is supplied by the **cystic artery**, which is usually a branch of the **right hepatic artery** (from the common hepatic artery). However, variations can occur in its origin and course.

The **bile duct** is formed by the union of the **cystic duct** (from the gallbladder) and the **common hepatic duct** (from the liver). It transports bile to the wall of the second part of the duodenum (the descending bit). Here, it is joined by the pancreatic duct at the **ampulla of Vater**, and opens into the duodenum at the duodenal papilla.

The maximum volume of the gallbladder is 30–60 mL. However, bile is concentrated within the bladder by the absorption of water, Na^+ and Cl^- into the gallbladder mucosa **(18b)**. Up to 12 hours of bile secretion is stored in concentrated form. Factors that cause contraction of the gallbladder are known as **cholagogues (18a)**. They include the entrance of food into the mouth, impulses from the **vagus nerve** and the secretion of **CCK**. Remember **CCK** is secreted in response to **fatty acids** and amino acids in the duodenum, as well as acid and Ca^{2+}.

The gallbladder starts emptying about 30 minutes after a meal is eaten. The walls contract rhythmically, and the **sphincter of Oddi** which guards the entrance to the duodenum relaxes. Relaxation of the sphincter of Oddi is assisted by: (1) peristaltic waves transmitted down the bile duct from the gallbladder, (2) cholecystokinin, and (3) intestinal peristaltic waves in the duodenum wall **(18c)**.

Answers
15. T F F T T
16. T T F F T
17. 1 – D, 2 – J, 3 – E, 4 – B, 5 – I, 6 – H, 7 – C, 8 – G, 9 – A, 10 – F
18. See explanation

19. Case study

An overweight 46-year-old smoker was admitted to the Emergency Department with a sudden onset of severe pain in the right upper quadrant of her abdomen, vomiting and fever. On palpation of her abdomen there was tenderness and guarding in the right upper quadrant, which became worse on inspiration. Ultrasound revealed a thickened gallbladder wall and pericholecystic fluid.

a. What are the risk factors for gallstones?

b. Why does this woman complain of pain in the shoulder?

c. What complications of this condition could arise?

EXPLANATION: GALLSTONES

Gallstones are most likely to affect you if you are:

- Fair
- Forty
- Fat
- Fertile
- Female

In other words, an obese middle-aged woman who has had several children (**remember the five 'Fs'**) **(19a)**. Smoking also increases the risk that gallstones will be symptomatic, although 50 per cent are not. Gallstones are generally more common in Europe and North America than in the rest of the world.

There are three types of stone: Ca^{2+} bilirubinate, cholesterol and mixed. Predisposing factors to their formation are: bile stasis, supersaturation of bile with cholesterol (due to excessive cholesterol excretion), and a mix of nucleation factors that favours stone formation. If gallstones become impacted in the gallbladder, cystic duct or bile duct they can cause a characteristic pain known as **biliary colic**. Pain may be referred to the **right shoulder** because the inflamed gallbladder may irritate the peritoneum covering the diaphragm **(19b)**. The skin of the shoulder is supplied by the same segments of the spinal cord that receive pain afferents from the diaphragm (**C3, C4**).

Complications of gallstones are numerous and depend on the location of the stone. Within the gallbladder, **acute cholecystitis** (inflammation and oedema of the gallbladder) may arise, empyema (pus in the gallbladder) and even perforation may occur **(19c)**. Organisms associated with cholecystitis are *Escherichia coli*, *Klebsiella* and *Streptococcus faecalis*. Repeated bouts of acute cholecystitis may result in chronic **cholecystitis**, with fibrosis of the gallbladder wall.

In the bile ducts, **obstructive jaundice**, **pancreatitis** or **cholangitis** (inflammation of the bile duct) may occur. And in the gut, there is a risk of gallstone ileus – a form of intestinal obstruction.

In this case it is likely the woman has acute cholecystitis because of the sudden onset, the fever and local peritonitis. The pain felt on inspiration is known as **Murphy's sign**. She would be treated initially with pain relief, fluids and antibiotics, then cholecystectomy.

Answers

19. See explanation

20. True or false? The insulin receptor

a. Contains two alpha subunits and two beta glycoprotein subunits
b. Has a tyrosine kinase domain on the intracellular ends of the alpha chain
c. Can be downregulated by a high concentration of insulin
d. Number is increased in the fed state
e. Does not always require autophosphorylation to exert its biological effects

21. Regarding the insulin receptor

a. It is a hexamer
b. The beta subunit binds insulin
c. Insulin receptor substrate mediates the actions of insulin
d. The beta subunit autophosphorylates on serine/threonine residues
e. Receptors may only be found on adipocytes

22. Label the indicated parts of the insulin receptor opposite

23. State whether the following metabolic processes are (1) increased, (2) decreased or (3) unaffected by insulin

Options

A. Lipolysis
B. Glucose transport into muscle cells
C. Glycogen breakdown
D. Conversion of glucose to fatty acids
E. Glucose uptake into brain cells
F. Active transport of amino acids into cells

EXPLANATION: THE INSULIN RECEPTOR AND THE EFFECTS OF INSULIN

The **insulin receptor** is a single polypeptide arranged into a tetramer of alpha and beta subunits linked by disulphide bonds (it belongs to a group of receptors called **tyrosine kinase receptors**). The receptors are found on **all tissues** including the liver. Insulin binds to the extracellular alpha subunits, which triggers **ATP** generation to cause **autophosphorylation** of the tyrosine residues on the membrane-spanning beta subunits. The beta subunits have a **tyrosine kinase domain,** and therefore following autophosphorylation they become activated tyrosine kinases which phosphorylate tyrosine residues on IRS, an important intracellular mediator of insulin's actions. The phosphorylation of IRS initiates its own catalytic activity and results in a **phosphorylation/dephosphorylation cascade** of intracellular proteins on serine and threonine residues which control the biological actions of insulin.

Insulin is essentially an anabolic hormone. It has stimulatory and inhibitory effects in the liver, muscle and adipose tissue – all insulin-sensitive tissues. In **hepatocytes**, insulin causes an increase in glycolysis, glycogen synthesis, fatty acid and triacylglycerol synthesis, and inhibits gluconeogenesis. In **adipocytes**, glucose uptake by GLUT-4 transporters is increased, as is lipogenesis. Insulin inactivates hormone-sensitive lipase so that breakdown of fat is inhibited. In **muscle**, again glucose uptake by GLUT-4 is increased, as are glycolysis, glycogen synthesis and protein synthesis. Glycogen degradation and proteolysis are inhibited. The brain and erythrocytes do not modify their glucose uptake in response to insulin.

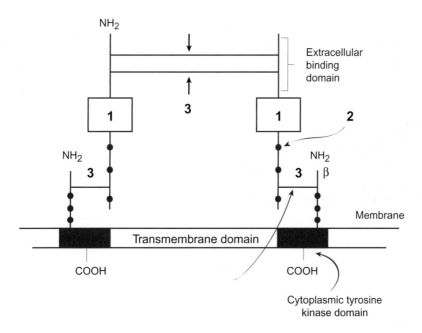

Answers

20. T F T F F
21. F F T F F
22. 1 – alpha subunit; 2 – cysteine residues; 3 – disulphide bridge
23. 1 – B, D, F; 2 – A, C; 3 – E

24. Regarding development of the liver

a. Growth begins in the middle of the third week of development
b. The liver is derived from ectodermal epithelium
c. The gallbladder and liver originate from the same liver bud
d. Haematopoiesis begins during the third week of development
e. The liver grows slowly during embryonic life

25. Regarding hepatobiliary development

a. The liver is derived from the midgut
b. The septum transversum is a mass of endodermal cells
c. The cranial part of the liver bud gives rise to the gallbladder
d. Bile formation begins in the 12th week
e. Biliary atresia results from the failure of the bile ducts to recanalize

26. Regarding the development of the pancreas

a. The pancreas develops in the 4th and 6th week of fetal life
b. The ventral bud migrates in front of the duodenum
c. The ventral bud and dorsal bud do not fuse until after birth
d. The accessory pancreatic duct is derived from the dorsal pancreatic bud
e. Insulin secretion begins at birth

EXPLANATION: DEVELOPMENT OF THE LIVER AND PANCREAS

The liver, the gallbladder and the bile duct all arise in the middle of the 3rd week to early in the 4th week of development from a **ventral outgrowth** of **endodermal epithelium** in the foregut called the liver bud or hepatic diverticulum.

The liver bud extends into the septum transversum, a mass of mesodermal cells between the pericardial cavity and the yolk sac. Septum transversum eventually forms the diaphragm and some ventral mesentery.

The liver bud actually **divides**, so that the cranial part forms the cells of the **liver parenchyma** and the caudal (inferior) part forms the **gallbladder** and **cystic duct**.

The liver grows very rapidly, intermingling with the umbilical and vitelline veins. Haematopoiesis begins during the 6th week, and bile formation by the hepatocytes begins in the 12th week.

The pancreas develops from two outgrowths of the endodermal epithelium, again in the foregut. They are the ventral pancreatic bud and the dorsal pancreatic bud.

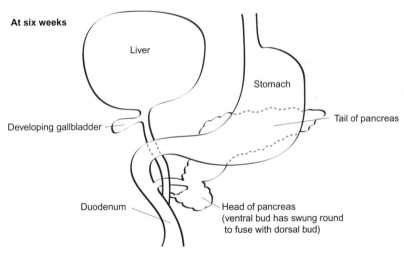

At six weeks

Liver

Stomach

Tail of pancreas

Developing gallbladder

Duodenum

Head of pancreas
(ventral bud has swung round
to fuse with dorsal bud)

The ventral pancreatic bud rotates and migrates round the back of the duodenum to join the dorsal bud, where the two buds fuse. Their respective ducts also fuse to form the main pancreatic duct that opens into the duodenum with the common bile duct. The accessory pancreatic duct which may be found in some individuals is actually a persistent part of the dorsal bud duct.

The ventral bud forms the head of the pancreas, whilst the dorsal bud forms the body and tail. Insulin is secreted during the 5th month of embryonic life.

Answers
24. T F T F F
25. F F F T T
26. T F F T F

27. True or false? Insulin

a. Is secreted into the bloodstream via the main pancreatic duct
b. Has intramolecular disulphide bridges
c. Is stored with C-peptide in granules
d. Cannot be broken down
e. Is formed from an inactive precursor

28. Insulin secretion is stimulated by

a. Adrenaline
b. A rise in blood glucose
c. Secretin
d. Glycerol
e. A rise in amino acid in the blood

29. In an oral glucose tolerance test, impaired glucose tolerance

a. Is demonstrated by a greater increase in plasma glucose than normal
b. Is demonstrated by a faster drop in plasma glucose to baseline than normal
c. Is caused by increased intestinal glucose absorption
d. Impairs the ability of the brain and red blood cells to take up glucose
e. Is diagnostic of diabetes mellitus

30. Regarding the oral glucose tolerance curve

a. On the adjacent graph, draw the glucose tolerance curve for: (i) a normoglycaemic person and (ii) a person with insulin-dependent diabetes
b. What is the normal range for fasting blood glucose?

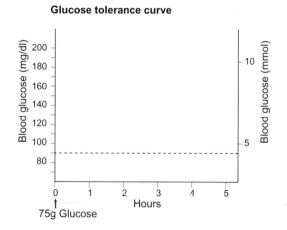

Glucose tolerance curve

EXPLANATION: INSULIN

Insulin is a **polypeptide hormone** produced by **beta-cells** of the **islets of Langerhans**. Beta-cells make up around 1 per cent of the mass of the pancreas. Insulin has **anabolic** effects on the **peripheral tissues**, promoting uptake of **glucose, protein synthesis, lipogenesis, glycogen synthesis** and **growth**.

Fifty-one amino acids are arranged into **two polypeptide chains** – A and B – linked by disulphide bridges. There are also intramolecular disulphide bridges between amino acid residues 6 and 11 of the A chain.

Insulin is synthesized from an inactive precursor. **Preproinsulin** has an N-terminal signal peptide cleaved in the rough endoplasmic reticulum to give proinsulin, which is transported to the Golgi where it is cleaved to give insulin and C-peptide which are stored in secretory granules in the cytosol. Secretion is by exocytosis on initiation by the appropriate stimulus.

Stimulate insulin secretion	Inhibit insulin secretion
Rise in blood glucose	Low blood glucose
Rise in plasma amino acids, especially arginine	Adrenaline (released in response to stress/trauma/extreme exercise)
Secretin (GI hormone released in response to ingestion of food)	
Glucagon	

The **oral glucose tolerance test** involves taking 75 g of glucose in 300 mL water after **fasting overnight**. Venous plasma glucose is measured before the drink and over the next 2 hours. An individual with **impaired glucose tolerance** will have a slightly higher than normal fasting plasma glucose, and their plasma glucose will be between 6.0 and 7.8 mmol/L 2 hours after intake **(30)**. If fasting plasma glucose is **>7.8 mmol** and plasma glucose remains **>11.1 mmol** 2 hours after intake, the individual is **diabetic**.

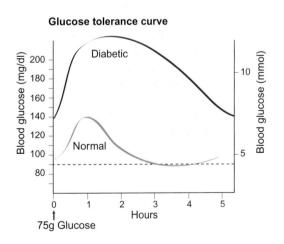

Glucose tolerance curve

31. Match the following features of acute liver failure to the causes listed below

Options

    A. Yellow skin
    B. Prone to bleeding
    C. Lethargy and drowsiness
    D. Low glomerular filtration rate
    E. Raised aspartate aminotransferase and alanine aminotransferase

    1. Failure of liver to synthesize proteins, depletion of factors II, VII, IX and X
    2. Circulation of excitatory amino acids, failure of liver to detoxify nitrogenous compounds
    3. Dysfunctional bilirubin metabolism
    4. Hepatocyte necrosis releases enzymes into bloodstream
    5. Shock due to a low circulating blood volume

32. Fatty changes to the liver

    a. Are caused by the accumulation of fat outside the liver
    b. May be caused by starvation
    c. May occur in pregnancy
    d. Are always irreversible
    e. Are usually lethal

GFR, glomerular filtration rate

EXPLANATION: LIVER FAILURE

Acute liver failure occurs when there has been damage to the majority of the **hepatocytes** in the liver, such that its functions are impaired. It may result from **metabolic damage**, severe **systemic shock** or as an **acute decline** in **chronic liver disease**. Acute liver failure has several key features.

Clinical **jaundice** is the yellowing of skin and sclerae caused by a high plasma **bilirubin** (above 50 μmol/L). This occurs in acute liver failure due to **dysfunctional bilirubin metabolism**. The liver is responsible for the **conjugation** and **secretion** of bilirubin in bile to the gut. Failure to do either results in accumulation of bilirubin in the blood.

Hepatic encephalopathy may be caused by acute liver failure. Features are progressive **drowsiness, lethargy** and eventually **coma**. It is caused by failure of the liver to detoxify nitrogenous compounds and the circulation of excitatory amino acids (which are not being deaminated in the liver).

Enzyme levels in the blood, such as **aspartate aminotransferase** and **alanine aminotransferase**, are useful clinical indicators of hepatocellular damage as they leak into the circulation.

Patients with liver failure may develop **kidney failure** (hepatorenal syndrome). Despite the almost normal histological appearance of the kidney, GFR is low, is as Na^+ concentration of the urine.

Fatty change is just one pattern of histological abnormality seen in the liver following damage. Triglycerides accumulate within the liver cells. It is most commonly seen when the liver is exposed to metabolic stress and alcohol. It is sublethal and, in the case of alcohol-induced fatty change, is reversible by abstinence.

The main causes of fatty liver are hypoxia, starvation, diabetes mellitus, alcohol, Reye's syndrome and pregnancy.

Other patterns of pathological response seen on damage to the liver are:

- Liver cell necrosis
- Fibrosis
- Cholestasis
- Storage of abnormal material.

Answers
31. 1 – B, 2 – C, 3 – A, 4 – E, 5 – D
32. F T T F F

33. Concerning hepatitis

a. Hepatitis A may lead to chronic liver disease
b. Hepatitis B is transmitted by the faecal–oral route
c. It is possible to carry hepatitis B and not show symptoms
d. It may be caused by the Epstein–Barr virus
e. Hepatitis C decreases the risk of hepatocellular carcinoma

34. Regarding acute hepatitis

a. Symptoms are low-grade pyrexia and malaise
b. It is not associated with jaundice
c. The cause is usually bacterial
d. Liver cells swell and become vacuolated
e. Recovery usually takes between 3 and 8 weeks

AST, aspartate aminotransferase; ALT, alanine aminotransferase

EXPLANATION: HEPATIC PATHOLOGY

There are **six** main patterns of **liver cell necrosis**:

1. Piecemeal necrosis   **2.** Massive necrosis   **3.** Zonal necrosis
4. Bridging necrosis   **5.** Councilman bodies   **6.** Spotty necrosis.

Spotty necrosis is usually seen with toxic damage and viral infection. In zonal necrosis, certain zones are affected by certain diseases, for example zone 3 is affected by paracetamol, whereas zone 1 is affected by phosphorous toxicity. Following **liver cell damage** there is **regeneration** of the liver cells to restore hepatic function. In cases of chronic damage, regeneration may be disturbed by **fibrosis**. ITO cells differentiate to secrete collagen in the space of Disse. This is the cause of **liver cirrhosis**.

Hepatitis is the term used to refer to **inflammatory diseases** of the liver. It may be acute or chronic. The main causes are **viral, autoimmune diseases, drug reactions** and **alcohol**. Viruses are a particularly common cause of hepatitis. Clinical features of acute hepatitis are **nausea, anorexia**, low-grade **pyrexia** and general **malaise**. **Jaundice** occurs a week to 10 days after the onset of symptoms. Serum **bilirubin** is usually raised, and levels of **ALT** and **AST** are very high early on in the disease. They fall as the liver regenerates itself. Recovery is within 3–8 weeks. The main hepatitis viruses are **A** and **E** – transmitted via the **faecal–oral** route – and **B, C** and **D**, which are transmitted via the **parenteral** route. Epstein–Barr virus and cytomegalovirus also cause hepatitis. The table below shows some of the important features of each virus:

Hepatitis	Virus type	Transmission route	Clinical features	Chronicity
A	RNA	Faecal–oral	Fever, malaise and nausea + vomiting within 2 weeks Jaundice 1 week later Nearly all patients fully recover Incubation 1–5 months	No
B	DNA	Parenteral, sexual, vertical (mother to baby)	Asymptomatic or similar to hepatitis A 95% fully recover 1% fulminant liver failure	Yes 5% chronic carriers ↑ risk of hepatocellular carcinoma
C	RNA	Parenteral	Acute infection is mild 20% jaundice 50% recover fully	Yes 50% chronic hepatitis ↑ risk of hepatocellular carcinoma
D	RNA. Requires presence of HBV to infect	Parenteral – seen in i.v. drug users, in particular	Illness is indistinguishable from hepatitis B Incubation 1 month	No
E	RNA	Faecal–oral	Mild infection associated with jaundice Mortality from fulminant liver failure is 1%	No

Answers
33. F F T T F
34. T F F T T

35. True or false? The following are histological features of liver cirrhosis

a. Councilman bodies
b. Fibrosis
c. Destruction of liver cells
d. Lymphoid cells in the portal tracts
e. Regeneration of hepatocytes to form nodules

36. Portal hypertension is caused by

a. Splenomegaly
b. Certain herbal teas
c. Liver cirrhosis
d. Portal vein thrombosis
e. Haemorrhoids

EXPLANATION: CIRRHOSIS OF THE LIVER

In **liver cirrhosis** the normal architecture of the liver is replaced by diffuse **nodules** of regenerated liver cells, separated by bands of **collagenous fibrosis**. Cirrhosis is **irreversible**. Two types are described histologically: micronodular, where the nodules are less than 3 mm in diameter, and macronodular, where the nodules are larger than 3 mm in diameter.

Alcohol is the most common cause of cirrhosis in the western world. It is associated with micronodules. Another common cause is chronic hepatitis (B and C), which is associated with macronodules. Less common causes are cystic fibrosis, biliary cirrhosis and autoimmune disease. The clinical features of liver cirrhosis are secondary to portal hypertension and liver cell failure.

The **portal vein accounts for 85 per cent of hepatic blood flow**. Obstruction to flow from the portal vein causes a build up of pressure in the portal vascular bed, resulting in **splenomegaly**, **ascites** and portosystemic anastamosis. Causes of portal hypertension can be pre-sinusoidal, sinusoidal or post-sinusoidal.

- **Pre-sinusoidal** – occlusion of the portal venous system before the portal tracts, for example portal vein thrombosis, predisposed to by local sepsis and polycythaemia.
- **Sinusoidal** – blockage in the sinusoids caused by hepatic diseases such as cirrhosis, portal tract fibrosis or polycystic disease of the liver.
- **Post-sinusoidal** – diseases that block central veins and venous branches. For example thrombosis of hepatic or central veins, scarring caused by alcohol abuse, cytotoxic drugs, ingestion of toxic alkaloids present in herbal teas, venous fibrosis caused by irradiation of the liver.

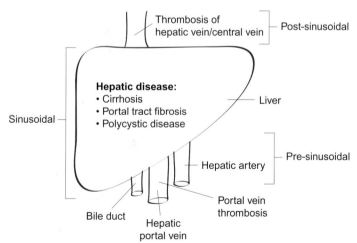

Budd–Chiari syndrome is caused by occlusion of the **hepatic vein**. Patients develop massive vascular congestion of the liver, which enlarges grossly. They also develop ascites very rapidly and jaundice. It can result in rapid death.

Answers
35. F T T F T
36. F T T T F

37. Regarding the pancreas

a. The head rests on the inferior vena cava
b. Pancreatic juice is secreted into the bile duct
c. The body lies at the level of L5
d. The pancreatic duct and common bile duct unite to form the ampulla
e. The tail lies between the layers of the splenorenal ligament

38. Pancreatic cancer

a. Usually affects the head of the pancreas
b. Causes obstructive jaundice
c. Is not associated with smoking
d. Presents with pain in the chest
e. Does not cause diabetes

39. Case study

A 45-year-old man is brought into the Emergency Department in agony, experiencing severe epigastric pain radiating through to the back, feeling nauseous and retching violently. The pain started 2 hours previously as he was returning from a meal out at a restaurant. On examination the man appeared jaundiced, was feverish and tachycardic.

Blood results showed a high white cell count, hyperglycaemia, a low plasma Ca^{2+} and a high level of amylase in the plasma.
a. What is the likely cause of this man's abdominal pain?
b. Why is he hyperglycaemic?
c. Why does he have a low plasma Ca^{2+}?

EXPLANATION: THE PANCREAS

The **pancreas** produces an **exocrine** secretion that enters the duodenum through the pancreatic duct and an endocrine secretion that enters the blood directly. The bile duct joins the pancreatic duct and carries only bile. The head of the pancreas is hugged by the C-curve of the duodenum. It rests on the inferior vena cava, the right renal artery and vein, and the left renal vein. The body lies at the level of L2.

Pancreatic cancer is the fifth most common cause of death in the western world. Cancers are invariably **ductal adenocarcinomas**. **Smoking** causes a two-fold increased risk, and 60 per cent of patients are male. Other risk factors are thought to be **high-fat, high-protein diets**, **alcohol** and **coffee**. Obstructive jaundice is caused by the compression of the bile duct by the tumour, together with dark urine and pale stools. Pancreatic cancer often **presents late** as an ill-defined pain radiating to the back, partially relieved by sitting up. **Exocrine** and **endocrine insufficiency** are also associated – diabetes mellitus or impaired glucose tolerance is present in one-third of patients. **Weight loss** (reflecting malabsorption, low dietary intake and depressed liver function), **steatorrhoea** and anorexia are also features. Surgical resection is the only hope for cure. The standard operation is **Whipple's procedure** – removal of the pancreas, distal stomach, duodenum, gallbladder and common bile duct, and then anastamoses between the jejunum and pancreatic remnant.

The man in the case study has **acute pancreatitis**, a very common reason for emergency admission to hospital **(39a)**. Major causes are **biliary tract disease** and heavy **alcohol** consumption. It may be precipitated by a **fat-rich meal**, causing **hyperlipidaemia**. The severity may range from mild oedema to severe necrosis and haemorrhage. The exact pathophysiology of pancreatitis remains unclear. It seems that a triggering factor causes premature activation of **pancreatic enzymes** within the pancreatic ducts, setting off a chain reaction of **cell necrosis** and **autodigestion**. Proteolytic enzyme release results in increased capillary permeability, protein exudation and oedema. The fluid loss causes hypovolaemic shock, which may be dangerous. Destruction of the islets of Langerhans leads to a transient **insulin deficiency** and therefore hyperglycaemia prevails **(39b)**. Liver function enzymes may be raised in the blood in alcoholic patients. **Plasma amylase**, a pancreatic digestive enzyme, is very high due to its release from damaged pancreatic cells. Another enzyme released is pancreatic lipase. It breaks down retroperitoneal fat to free fatty acids, which then absorb Ca^{2+} to form insoluble Ca^{2+} salts. This is what causes the low plasma Ca^{2+} **(39c)**.

Answers

37. T F F T T
38. T T F F F
39. See explanation

40. True or false? Bilirubin

a. Is formed from the degradation of haemoglobin
b. Is transported free in the plasma
c. Is conjugated in the kidney
d. May undergo enterohepatic recirculation
e. Is excreted in the urine as stercobilinogen

41. Jaundice

a. Is characterized by a high concentration of bilirubin in the blood
b. Causes itching of the skin
c. Is a sign of liver disease
d. May be caused by gallstones impacted in the bile duct
e. Is cured by removal of the gallbladder

42. Define the following terms

a. First pass metabolism
b. Phase I reaction
c. Phase II reaction

sER, smooth endoplasmic reticulum; GB, gallbladder; RBC, red blood cell

EXPLANATION: JAUNDICE AND DRUG METABOLISM

The bilirubin pathway is shown on page 102.

Jaundice is caused by **abnormalities** either in **bilirubin metabolism** in the liver or in bilirubin **excretion**, resulting in an elevation in its level in the blood (30–60 μmol/L). It is characterized by yellowing of the skin and cornea, and pruritus (itching). The liver normally conjugates bilirubin to make it more water soluble and to ensure it is excreted in the urine. If the liver is unable to do this, bilirubin builds up in the plasma, causing **prehepatic jaundice**:

- Haemolysis – too much bilirubin is formed
- Gilbert's syndrome – abnormalities in bilirubin handling by liver
- Crigler–Najjar syndrome – liver cells have defect in the enzyme that conjugates bilirubin.

Cholestatic/obstructive jaundice is caused by a blockage in the excretion of conjugated bilirubin from the liver to the small intestine. Conjugated bilirubin builds up in the blood. Since it is water soluble, it is excreted in the urine and turns it dark. However, the stools are pale since bile is absent from the faeces. Cholestasis may be either **intrahepatic** (hepatitis, cirrhosis, pregancy-associated, hereditary enzyme defects) or **extrahepatic** (gallstone in the bile duct, carcinoma of head of pancreas).

Some drugs are **inactivated** in the **liver**. They are removed from the portal circulation and **metabolized**. Therefore the concentration of the drug reaching the systemic circulation is much less than that in the portal vein. This is known as **first pass metabolism (42a)**. Examples of drugs that undergo first pass metabolism include aspirin, lignocaine, morphine and propanolol.

The disadvantages of first pass metabolism are that a much larger dose of the drug is required orally than via other routes. Also, there is a marked individual variation in the extent to which drugs are metabolized like this, so there is some unpredictability in determining how much drug will reach the systemic circulation.

Metabolism of drugs in the liver involves two kinds of reaction: **phase I and phase II**. **Phase I** is usually **oxidation**, **reduction** or **hydrolysis (42b)**. The products of the reaction usually have a reduced biological activity compared with the original drug, but may be more toxic. The aim of this reaction is to give the drug a reactive chemical handle, so that it may proceed to phase II.

Phase II reaction involves the **conjugation** of a drug molecule with a suitably reactive handle **(42c)**. Conjugation is basically the attachment of a substituent group. The new conjugate is **pharmacologically inactive** and more water soluble than its precursor, therefore it is readily excreted in the urine.

Answers

40. T F F T F
41. T T T T F
42. See explanation

43. The following drugs undergo first pass metabolism. True or false?

a. Sulphonureas
b. Aspirin
c. Oral contraceptive pill
d. Propanalol
e. Metronidazole

44. The following drugs are hepatotoxic

a. Halothane
b. Androgens
c. Paracetamol
d. Alcohol
e. Isoniazid

45. Theme – chemical pathology of the liver. Match the following laboratory test results to their respective indications

Options

A. Liver cell necrosis
B. Cholestasis
C. Alcohol-induced damage
D. Chronic liver disease
E. Acute hepatitis

1. Raised serum albumin
2. Extremely high aspartate aminotransferase
3. Raised alkaline phosphatase
4. Prolonged prothrombin time
5. Raised gamma glutamyl transpeptidase

The bilirubin pathway (see Question 40, page 100).

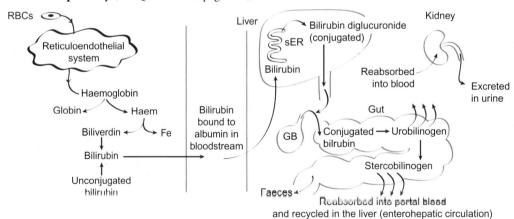

GGT, gamma glutamyl transferase; AST, aspartate aminotransferase

EXPLANATION: HEPATOTOXIC DRUGS

Many **drugs** may cause **liver cell damage**, which presents as hepatitis or cholestasis.

Paracetamol and isoniazid cause **hepatocyte necrosis** due to their highly reactive metabolites, which may form covalent or non-covalent bonds with cell components. Covalent bonds are formed with DNA, proteins, lipids and carbohydrates. Non-covalent interactions include lipid peroxidation, generation of toxic free radicals and reactions depleting glutathione (an important participant in phase II reactions). **Chlorpromazine** and androgen steroids cause a different type of liver cell damage which results in **obstructive jaundice**. Some drugs cause an **autoimmune reaction** in the liver. **Halothane** is thought to damage liver cells by this mechanism.

Paracetamol toxicity is clinically very **important**, as it is a common cause of death from self-poisoning. Paracetamol is usually very safe when taken in the correct doses. Normally it is metabolized in the liver by two routes of conjugation. However, in massive doses the enzymes catalysing the conjugation reactions are saturated, and the toxic reactive intermediate in the pathway accumulates (*N*-acetyl-*p*-benzoquinoneimine). The **intermediate** causes **liver cell death**. Fulminant **liver failure** usually develops within 36–48 hours due to massive necrosis.

The liver function tests and their meanings are listed below.

Test	Normal range	Results	Interpretation
Serum bilirubin	<17 µmol/L	↑ unconjugated ↑ conjugated	Pre-hepatic jaundice Intrahepatic or extrahepatic cholectasis
Alkaline phosphatase enzyme found in bone, gut, placenta and liver, especially bile canalicular region	90–300 iu/L	Raised	Bone disease or liver disease: particularly indicative or cholestasis because enzyme is released proximal to the obstruction and refluxes into blood
GGT	Men: up to 51 iu/L Women: up to 33 iu/L	Raised	GGT synthase is stimulated by alcohol and other drugs
Albumin	30–55 g/L	Lowered	Albumin has long half-life (21 days) therefore is a good indicator of chronic liver disease affecting synthesis
AST found in liver and muscle	<50 iu/L	Very high Moderately high	Severe hepatis: necrosis Membrane damage, no necrosis
Prothrombin time	Control ± 4 s	Longer than normal	Prothrombin time depends on synthesis of clotting factors. These have short half-lives. Good indicator of acute hepatitis because affected quickly

Answers

43. F T T T F
44. T T T T T
45. 1 – D, 2 – A, 3 – B, 4 – E, 5 – C

46. Explain the mechanism by which the following occur in liver failure

    a. Ascites
    b. Gynaecomastia
    c. Hypoglycaemia

47. The following are signs of chronic liver disease. True or false?

    a. Exophthalmia
    b. Flapping tremor
    c. Ascites
    d. Aphthous ulcers
    e. Spider naevi

48. Theme – the pancreas. Match the following exocrine pancreatic secretions to their correct action

Options

A. Pancreatic lipase
C. Bicarbonate
E. Phospholipase A$_2$

B. Trypsin
D. Pancreatic alpha-amylase
F. Elastase

1. Removes fatty acid from carbon 2 of phospholipid
2. Removes fatty acids from carbon 1 and 3 in triacylglycerides
3. Digests proteins and polypeptides
4. Neutralizes gastric acid to pH 6 or 7
5. Breaks down elastin
6. Breaks down starch

49. The following factors increase pancreatic exocrine secretion

    a. Sympathetic stimulation
    c. Gastrin
    e. Vagal stimulation

    b. Secretin
    d. Somatostatin

EXPLANATION: CONSEQUENCES OF LIVER FAILURE (QUESTIONS 46 AND 47)

The consequences of liver failure are all related to the deterioration of the main functions of the liver.

Ascites is related to a reduction in the synthesis of plasma proteins such as albumin and clotting factors **(46a)**. Hypoalbuminaemia causes a loss of **oncotic pressure** across the capillary walls. This is the osmotic force exerted by plasma proteins to pull water into the blood. With a loss of this force, fluid escapes from the circulation into the interstitial space, resulting in peripheral oedema. Fluid accumulating in the **peritoneal cavity** is known as ascites.

With liver failure, hormones tend to accumulate in the bloodstream.

- **Aldosterone** – Na^+ and **water retention**
- **Oestrogen** – **gynaecomastia** in men and loss of secondary sex characteristics **(46b)**
- **Insulin** – reduced **glycogen breakdown**, impaired **gluconeogenesis**, and therefore **lowered blood glucose** **(46c)**.

Cirrhosis or chronic liver disease resulting in irreversible changes to the liver has a variety of physical signs that can be seen in the patient on close examination. **Spider naevi** appear on the surface of the skin as a central arteriole from which a series of smaller vessels branch. They are formed by local vascular dilation due to high oestrogen levels and commonly occur on the neck, face and dorsa of the hands. Other physical signs are **clubbing** of the finger nails, a **flapping tremor** caused by hepatic encephalopathy, **loss of body hair**, **bruising** due to deficiency in clotting factors, a swollen abdomen due to the fluid retention of **ascites**, and **xanthelasmata** – cholesterol deposition around the eyelids. Aphthous ulcers are a feature of inflammatory bowel disease; exophthalmia is seen in hyperthyroidism.

EXPLANATION: PANCREATIC SECRETION (i)

Pancreatic juice contains:

- Cations: Na^+, K^+, Ca^{2+}, Mg^{2+}
- Anions: HCO_3^-, Cl^-, SO_4^{2-}, HPO_4^{2-}

The **digestive secretions** of the pancreas are formed in the **acini**, rather similar to the acini of the salivary glands and secreted into a **network of ducts** that meet to form the **main pancreatic duct**. This duct empties into the duodenum. The pancreas secretes around 1 L of fluid per day; at rest this fluid is plasma-like, but it becomes more alkaline at higher flow rates. This is because as it travels through the ducts, Cl^- is exchanged for HCO_3^- ions. At higher flow rates there is less time for the exchange to take place. Pancreatic secretions **neutralize** the **acid chyme** from the stomach in the duodenum to establish the optimum pH (6–7) at which pancreatic enzymes act.

Answers

46. See explanation
47. F T T F T
48. 1 – E, 2 – A, 3 – B, 4 – C, 5 – F, 6 – E
49. F T T F T

50. Concerning pancreatic enzymes

a. They are released in precursor form to prevent autodigestion
b. Pancreatic amylase differs in action to salivary amylase
c. Trypsinogen activates the proteases
d. Enterokinase is secreted via the main pancreatic duct
e. Pancreatic amylase is activated by Cl⁻ ions

51. True or false. Cystic fibrosis

a. Affects 1 in 25 in white populations
b. Is characterized by absent or deficient pancreatic enzymes
c. Results in a deficiency in fat-soluble vitamins
d. Is caused by a defective sodium ion transporter
e. May affect the bronchi

CCK, cholecystokinin

EXPLANATION: PANCREATIC SECRETION (ii)

Pancreatic secretion has a **cephalic** phase during which secretion is stimulated by vagal nerve activity.

In the **gastric** phase, the release of **gastrin** from the antrum stimulates secretion, but the major stimulus is in the **intestinal** phase. Chyme entering the duodenum stimulates a bicarbonate- and enzyme-rich secretion of fluid from the pancreas, as a result of the actions of **secretin** and **CCK** released from the mucosa of the small intestine. Sympathetic stimulation inhibits pancreatic secretion.

THE ENZYMES   The table below summarizes the pancreatic enzymes and their actions.

Digestive enzyme	Activator	Substrate	Action
Trypsin(ogen)	Enteropeptidase	Proteins/polypeptides	Cleaves peptide bonds adjacent to arginine or lysine
Chymotrypsin(ogen)	Trypsin	Proteins/polypeptides	Cleaves peptide bonds adjacent to arginine or lysine
(Pro)elastase	Trypsin	Elastin	Cleaves bonds next to aliphatic amino acids
Carboxypeptidase A and B	Trypsin	Proteins/polypeptides	Cleaves C-terminal amino acids
Ribonuclease	–	RNA	Cleaves to release nucleotides
Deoxyribonuclease	–	DNA	Releases nucleotides
Co-lipase	Trypsin	Fat droplets	Binds to make anchor for lipase
Pancreatic lipase	–	Triglycerides	Hydrolysis to free fatty acids and glycerol
Phospholipase A_2	Trypsin	Phospholipids	Release fatty acis and lysophospholipids
Pancreatic alpha-amylase	Cl$^-$	Starch	Hydrolysis of α 1–4 linkages

Protease precursors (**chymotrypsinogen**, procarboxypeptidases) are activated by **trypsin**, which is formed from **trypsinogen** by the action of enterokinase. Enterokinase is not secreted in the pancreatic duct but found on the brush border of the small intestine mucosa. Pancreatic **amylase** splits alpha 1,4 linkages between **starch residues**. **Lipases** are also present to act on triglycerides and phospholipids.

Cystic fibrosis affects 1 in 2500 white people. It is an autosomal recessive disorder characterized by recurrent chest infections and exocrine pancreatic insufficiency. A defective chloride ion channel in the epithelial cells causes decreased secretion of sodium and water. The result is the production of a particularly thick and viscous mucus that cannot be easily cleared from the lungs and that blocks the pancreatic ducts. With time, the pancreatic acini atrophy. The median age of survival is 30 years.

Answers
50. T F F F T
51. F T T F T

52. Concerning the endocrine pancreas

a. Beta cells make up 75 per cent of the cells in the islets
b. Alpha cells secrete somatostatin
c. Islets of Langerhans are most plentiful in the head of the pancreas
d. Insulin is complexed with zinc in beta cell granules
e. Ca^{2+} ion influx into the beta cell triggers insulin exocytosis

53. True or false? Glucagon

a. Is secreted by beta cells in the islets of Langerhans
b. Causes ketone body formation
c. Mediates its effects through a cAMP-dependent kinase
d. Is secreted in response to adrenaline
e. Is high in the plasma during the fed state

54. Hyperglycaemia

a. Is diagnosed at a fasting blood glucose of >7.8 mmol/L
b. Causes polyuria
c. Might be caused by an insulinoma
d. Increases sensitivity to insulin
e. May be managed through diet alone

cAMP, cyclic adenosine monophosphate; RBC, red blood cell

EXPLANATION: INSULIN AND GLUCOSE CONTROL

The **endocrine portion** of the pancreas makes up just **2 per cent** of the organ. **Endocrine cells** are localized in **islets of Langerhans**.

Insulin is produced by **beta cells**, **glucagon** is produced by **alpha cells** and **somatostatin** is produced by **delta cells**. Insulin is stored in **vesicles** in beta cells complexed with **zinc**. It has a biphasic pattern of secretion. No matter what the stimulatory factor on the beta cell is, ultimately it is the intracellular rise in Ca^{2+} ions that causes insulin exocytosis.

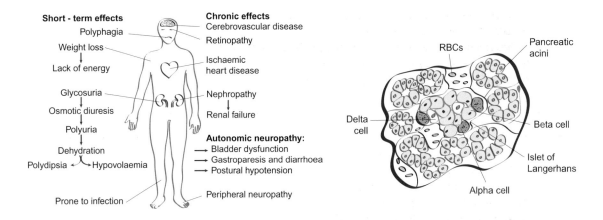

Glucagon has **antagonistic** effects to **insulin** and is therefore a catabolic hormone. Stimulants of its release from alpha cells are: **falling blood glucose** concentration, **amino acids**, **catecholamines** and **gut hormones**. Glucogon binds to a G protein coupled receptor on its target cells, which stimulates the production of cAMP, which in turn activates appropriate protein kinases to phosphorylate intracellular proteins. Deficiency of glucagon does not normally cause a problem since other catabolic hormones can perform its function.

Hyperglycaemia is an excess of glucose in the blood. It is usually caused by **insulin** deficiency and/or insulin **resistance** (diabetes mellitus). However, it can occur in rare cases of glucagonoma – a tumour of the pancreas. High blood glucose has a variety of detrimental effects on the body, outlined in the diagram opposite.

Glucose control in diabetes is generally managed through **diet** and **insulin replacement** therapy. Dietary measures include switching from foods with readily assimilable sugars to slow-release carbohydrates, snacking regularly (if taking insulin) and eating a high-fibre, low saturated fat diet

Answers
52. T F F T T
53. F T T T F
54. T T F F T

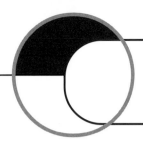

Index